FOUL PLAY

Drug Abuse in Sports

FOUL PLAY

Drug Abuse in Sports

Tom Donohoe
Neil Johnson

Basil Blackwell

© Tom Donohoe and Neil Johnson 1986

First published 1986
Reprinted 1987

Basil Blackwell Ltd
108 Cowley Road, Oxford OX4 1JF, UK

Basil Blackwell Inc.
432 Park Avenue South, Suite 1503,
New York, NY 10016, USA

BRITISH LIBRARY CATALOGUING IN PUBLICATION DATA

Donohoe, Tom
  Foul play : drug abuse in sports.
  1. Drugs and sports
  I. Title   II. Johnson, Neil
  362.2′ 93′ 088796   GV706.8

  ISBN 0-631-14844-2

LIBRARY OF CONGRESS CATALOGING IN PUBLICATION DATA

Donohoe, Tom.
  Foul play.

  Bibliography : p.
  Includes indexes.
  1. Doping in sports.   2. Athletes—Drug use.
  I. Johnson, Neil.   II. Title.
  RC1230.D66   1986   362.2′ 93′ 088796   85-30624
  ISBN 0-631-14844-2

Printed in the USA

CONTENTS

v

FOREWORD

In 1981 I was honoured to be asked to address the International Olympic Congress in West Germany. As the host chairman of the Athletic Committee of the IOC, I spoke of the many problems facing the competitors in the Olympic movement. Of the problems I talked about that day, none assumed more importance than the use and abuse of drugs in sport.

The Olympic movement and numerous governing bodies of sport have often spent inordinate amounts of time looking into futile arguments of whether it is morally possible for Olympic competitors to uphold the tradition of the movement and make financial gains from their talents. A shift from this debate to that on drug abuse, which has eaten insidiously into the fabric of sport, is long overdue. I therefore welcome the publication of this excellent book with its sane and timely discussion on the abuse of drugs by athletes. Nothing stands more overtly against the basis of Olympism than the use of illegal substances in order to achieve victory. It is the very antithesis of fair play.

Sebastian Coe
April 1986

Preface

It is our hope that this book will be read by everyone with an interest in the future of modern sport. As scientists we were amazed by the way athletes abuse drugs to improve performance when even a cursory examination of the research shows that, in many cases, their use is not justified. The 'benefits' are often obtained at the expense of frightening risks, both medical and professional, yet drug abuse will probably continue unabated for as long as sport remains. As sportsmen this realisation led us away from a purely scientific appraisal of the problem to an investigation of the many wide-reaching social and political implications. These are the basic ingredients of an international scandal; one whose practices have advanced along with those of biological science to the extent that today most top athletes believe it is impossible to reach the top without using drugs.

In describing the nature and effects of doping substances to the layman we have evaluated the findings of current scientific research. The findings are sometimes contradictory (though hopefully not confusing!), often surprising and always fascinating. Scientific knowledge is a legacy from which everyone should benefit, so we hope this book does something to bridge the ever-widening gulf between lay and scientific opinion. By taking a rational, objective approach we also hope to put this enormous problem into some sort of perspective. This book reveals how drugs have corrupted the whole of sport, from school playing field to Olympic stadium. While we may not like to think of top sportsmen and women as being manipulated or prepared with drugs, this is often the reality. If there is any meaning left in the expression 'fair play' then this chemical war must stop.

Tom Donohoe
Neil Johnson
1985

ACKNOWLEDGEMENTS

In writing this book we are indebted to a large number of people whose assistance has been invaluable. Our thanks are due mainly to Tony Donohoe who edited, and commented on, the original draft. In addition we would like to thank Kim Pickin, of Basil Blackwell, who provided further editorial assistance. We would also like to acknowledge the co-operation of the following individuals and organisations and apologise for any omissions:

Amateur Fencing Association (Raymond Crawford, Medical Officer); Amateur Swimming Association (A. Williams, Chief Administrative Assistant); Arsenal Football Club; British Amateur Gymnastics Association (Diane Windsor); British Board of Boxing Control (R. L. Clarke, General Secretary); British Cycling Federation (Bryan Wotton, Racing Secretary); British Judo Association; Chelsea College Drug Testing Centre, University of London (Professor Arnold Beckett; Dr. David Cowan); Coventry City Football Club (George Dalton, physiotherapist); English Olympic Wrestling Association; The Football Association (Ted Croker, General Secretary); International Amateur Athletics Federation (Robert Helmick, Honorary Secretary); International Olympic Committee (Prince Alexandre de Merode, Chairman of Medical Division); International Tennis Federation (Shirley Woodhead, Acting General Secretary); Professor David Lamb, Ohio State University; Manchester United Football Club; Professor Arnold J.

ACKNOWLEDGEMENTS

Mandell, University of California, San Diego; Dave McVay; National Collegiate Athletic Association (Eric Zemper, Research Co-ordinator); John Rodda, *The Guardian*; The British Sports Council; Sports Council for Northern Ireland (Con O'Callaghan); Sports Council for Scotland; Squash Rackets Association (R. I. Morris, Chief Executive); Cliff Temple; Tottenham Hotspur Football Club (Peter Shreeve, Manager); Union of European Football Associations (Hans Bangerter, General Secretary); United States Olympic Committee (Bob Beeten, Manager, Clinical Services); University of Birmingham, Sports Documentation Centre, University Library; University of Nottingham, Department of Psychology; Wolverhampton Wanderers Football Club (P. G. Redfern, Club Secretary); Women's Amateur Athletic Association (Ms. M. Hartman, Honorary Secretary).

PICTURE ACKNOWLEDGEMENTS

We would like to thank the following for permission to reproduce photographs in this book. Should appropriate acknowledgement not have been made in any instance, this will be corrected in a future edition and we apologise for the omission.

Plates 1, 8, 12, 13 © BBC Hulton Picture Library; Plates 2, 3, 7, 9, 15, 17 © All-Sport; Plates 4, 14 © Tony Duffy, All-Sport; Plate 10 from MacCallum's *Textbook of Pathology*, W. B. Saunders, Philadelphia; Plate 6 from Professor Arnold J. Mandell; Plate 5 from *Purnell's New Encyclopedia of Association Football*, 1978, Purnell; Plate 11 from Money, J. and Ehrhardt, A.A. *Man and Woman, Boy and Girl* © 1973 the Johns Hopkins University Press, Baltimore, Maryland; Plate 16 © Sport and General Press Agency.

We would also like to thank those people who helped to find pictures; in particular Dave Taylor, Robert Pratten, The Wellcome Museum of Medical Science (Ms. S. Aspinall), Elizabeth Lake and Julia Mosse.

1

INTRODUCTION

The overwhelming majority of athletes I know would do anything, and take anything, short of killing themselves to improve
athletic performance.
Harold Connolly, 1956 Olympic hammer-throw champion,
testifying to a United States Senate Committee in 1973

Speaking at the Olympic Congress at Baden–Baden in 1981, on
behalf of athletes, Sebastian Coe, the 1500m gold medallist in
the 1980 Games, said:

We consider this [doping] to be the most shameful abuse
of the Olympic ideal: we call for the life ban of offending
athletes; we call for the life ban of coaches and the so-called
doctors who administer this evil.

This worthy sentiment is far removed from the tough, competitive world of modern sport where the use of drugs has become
firmly entrenched. Much of the recent controversy concerning
doping in sport has surrounded the use of anabolic steroids, but
the sheer range of other drugs and 'potions' used by athletes to
improve performance has reached dramatic proportions. The
legislation and detection methods available are continually
struggling to keep up with what the athlete is using.
The word doping stems from the Dutch word 'dop', which
was the name of a type of brandy made from grape skins in
South Africa. Its use was then broadened to include other

1

stimulating beverages. By the turn of the century, the term 'doping' was used to describe the administration of treatments to horses or greyhounds usually to *reduce* their chance of winning, and hence to influence the outcome of bets. In contemporary use, the expression has been applied to the use of any substance that alters the performance of a competitor in a sporting event. However, doping now refers to the use of substances to *improve* sporting performance.

Considering the prevalence of doping, it is surprising that little is known about the effects of these drugs on performance and more importantly, on long-term health. Popular opinion concerning doping in sport is often distorted, exaggerated, or sometimes even wrong. These misinformed views often extend to individuals who are either supplying, advocating the use, or actually taking the drugs, in other words the trainers, coaches and athletes themselves. Consequently, athletes commonly use dosages *far* in excess of those employed in medical practice, which may lead to many adverse psychological and physical side effects.

Performance-enhancing substances have been used by athletes for well over 2000 years. At the Ancient Olympic Games, athletes had special diets and ingested various substances believed to augment their physical capabilities. Charmis, the winner of the 200m sprint in the Olympic Games of 668 BC, was said to have a special diet of dried figs[1]. In Ancient Egypt the rear hooves of an Abyssinian ass, ground up, boiled in oil, and flavoured with rose petals and rose hips was the prescription recommended to improve performance[2]. There are many instances of stimulant substances being used through the ages. For example, Roman gladiators or knights in medieval jousts used stimulants after sustaining injury in order to continue the combat. However, it is only in recent times with improvements in chemical technology that a massive acceleration in the incidence of doping in sport has occurred.

Doping has been defined as the administration to, or the use by, a competing athlete of any substance foreign to the body or of any physiological substance taken in abnormal quantity or by

2

an abnormal route of entry in to the body, with the sole intention of increasing performance in an artificial and unfair manner[3]. The remainder of this chapter looks at some sporting events where competitors have been suspected of having, or were actually found to have taken, some form of dope. It is not intended to be a complete record, but rather to demonstrate the range of drugs used by athletes. It also illustrates how interpretation of the term 'doping' has changed, particularly over the last 30 years[4].

While swimmers in the 1865 Amsterdam canal races were suspected of taking some form of dope, the racing cyclists appeared to be the prime offenders of the time, especially participants in the infamous 6-day cycle races. Lasting from Monday morning to Saturday evening, these races placed extreme physical and psychological demands on the riders; consequently many of them turned to various stimulant preparations. The French used a mixture known as 'Caffeine Houdes' while the Belgians sucked on sugar cubes dipped in ether. The riders' black coffee was 'boosted' with extra caffeine and peppermint, and as the race progressed the mixture was spiked with increasing doses of cocaine or strychnine. Brandy was also frequently added to cups of tea. Following the sprint sequences of the race, nitroglycerine capsules were often given to the cyclists to ease breathing difficulties. The individual 6-day races were eventually replaced by two-man races, but the doping continued unabated. Since drugs such as heroin or cocaine were widely taken in these tournaments without supervision, it was perhaps likely that fatalities would occur.

It has been suggested that one of the first doping-related deaths was that of Arthur Linton, who was reported to have died in 1886, during the Bordeaux to Paris race, after having apparently been given an overdose by his trainer. It now appears that the facts somehow became distorted over the years. Arthur Linton won the Bordeaux to Paris race and according to *The Cycling World Illustrated* of 1896, actually died in July 1896 of an illness that was diagnosed as typhoid fever. According to Bryan Wotton, secretary of the British Cycling

3

Federation, Linton, a Welsh champion, was one of several riders trained by 'Choppy' Warburton[5]. It is known that many of these riders were given *strychnine* during competition. Warburton was eventually banned for life, but the precise reasons for the ban are not known. It is likely that Linton was doped, and in the long term, this may have caused his ill-health. While the cause of death was apparently typhoid fever, the use of dope may have eventually contributed to Linton's death. At very low doses, strychnine has a stimulant effect, but at higher doses is extremely poisonous.

Cycling was only one of the endurance sports where the advantages of doping were exploited. Boxers regularly used a range of drugs as stimulants and to ease pain. Drinks of honey and brandy, sips of dilute solutions of aromatic spirits of ammonia, or even strychnine tablets were taken during the fights. Some fighters were also massaged with an ointment mixture containing cocaine, to provide some surface anaesthesia. Heroin was widely used by boxers for its anaesthetic and stimulating properties. It has been suggested that many of the apparently punch-drunk fighters of the late nineteenth century may have been heroin addicts. The final remedy to keep the fighter 'alert' was the running of a flame down the back.

At the turn of this century, boxing and other sports were increasingly involved with money prizes and gambling. The large sums involved in the horse racing business also created the necessary incentives for doping. Bribery and corruption became a major problem and horses were often doped with cocaine. In particular, several Americans were suspected of doping horses at races in France. In Britain, George Lambton, the trainer of Lord Derby's horses, even doped his own animals to prove to the Jockey Club that something had to be done about such practices. Doping was actually forbidden in 1903, but it was difficult to prove without appropriate tests. It was first demonstrated in 1910 by Professor Fraenkel, when a saliva test on a horse in Austria revealed the presence of drugs. Two years later, Bourbon Rose, first in the Gold Cup at Maisons-Laffitte, was disqualified after failing a dope test. However,

4

'positive' doping was becoming a bigger problem in athletics. In the 1904 Olympic Marathon at St. Louis, an Englishman named Thomas Hicks, who was running for the USA, was helped to victory with the use of brandy and possibly strychnine. Similarly, Dorando Pietri was also suspected of taking strychnine in the 1908 Olympic Marathon in London. Pietri collapsed a few metres from the finishing line and was helped to his feet by several spectators, but their assistance caused his subsequent disqualification.

The use of drugs, particularly in professional sports, continued uncontrolled into the twentieth century. In Britain, the first Dangerous Drugs Act of 1920 required that drugs such as opium and cocaine were available only on prescription. While this reduced the availability of many drugs, it was still possible to buy many drugs (e.g. laudanum) 'over the counter'. The production of amphetamine-like stimulants in the thirties heralded a whole new era of doping in sport and the development of stimulants flourished during the Second World War. These drugs were given to troops to promote arousal and delay the onset of fatigue but they also produced a lack of judgement which made them unsuitable for use by air crews.

Following the war, sport began to tempt many people with bigger prize money, and stimulant use soared. Rumours of doping abounded in the popular press whenever a particular individual or team suddenly began to achieve better results. This was certainly the case for professional soccer players in England, some of whom were reported to be taking 'monkey gland' extracts, or other 'pep-pills', as stimulants. There was also a continuation of drug abuse in boxing and cycling, the extent of which was highlighted in the 1940s and 1950s by several deaths due to overdosing. Amazingly, no surprise was expressed outside the immediate circles concerned. This was particularly unusual in view of the outcry at suspected doping which took place at the 1952 Helsinki Olympics and the 1956 Melbourne Olympics. Doctors alleged that one competitor at the Melbourne Games showed spasms characteristic of strychnine poisoning. In 1958, the American Medical Association

5

surveyed over 400 trainers and coaches and found that over a third had had personal experience of stimulants and only 7 per cent knew nothing about them.

The 1960 Olympics in Rome was the scene of unprecedented drug-taking. This was highlighted by the death of the 23-year-old Danish cyclist Knud Jensen on the opening day while competing in the 100km team time-trial races. While the official verdict cited sunstroke as the cause of death, the autopsy revealed that Jensen had taken the stimulant amphetamine and also nicotinyl tartrate to increase the blood supply to his muscles. Two of his colleagues were also taken to hospital in a toxic condition. Another team-mate, Jorgen Jorgensen, also collapsed with mild sunstroke. There were *no* rules against doping in the Olympics at this time but Jensen's death highlighted a growing problem, and the International Olympic Committee (IOC) came under increasing pressure, particularly from the International Federation of Sports Medicine, to take immediate action.

In 1963 France introduced the first anti-doping law and was followed by Belgium two years later. However, this did not prevent widespread drug use at the Tokyo Olympics in 1964. The only sport investigated in Tokyo was cycling where riders were checked for signs of injections, 'frisked' on the starting line for tablets or capsules, and urine samples were taken after some of the races. Many urine samples were actually *blue* in colour due to the use of various drugs. However, only a few 'inoffensive' drugs were reported. Perhaps more importantly, many athletes were said to be 'unco-operative', which prompted several of the medical officers to send a letter of complaint to the IOC President Avery Brundage. A year later at the Tour of Britain Milk Race, three Spanish riders and an English cyclist were found to have traces of the stimulant amphetamine in their urine samples.

The extent of amphetamine abuse was not fully appreciated until tests conducted on Belgian cyclists in 1965 revealed that over 37 per cent of professionals and 23 per cent of amateurs were taking amphetamines. Furthermore, reports from Italy,

6

using fairly crude testing procedures, indicated that 46 per cent of all professional cyclists registered positive in dope tests. Further studies in Italy suggested that the problem was not confined to cycling. In 1961, Professor Ottani claimed that 88 per cent of Italian First Division soccer players used drugs in both games and training. However, dope testing of a random sample of players was carried out at the 1966 World Cup in England, in which Italy played, but nothing was found.

Cycling received more attention when, in 1966, the first five men to finish in the professional world road-race championships all refused to take a doping test. These included the world-famous cyclists Jacques Anquetil, Raymond Poulidor and Rudi Altig. They were suspended by the International Cycling Union, but were all reinstated a few months later. Anquetil later admitted taking stimulants during races. He said 'Everyone in cycling dopes himself and those who claim they don't are liars'. At the 1967 Pan-America Games in Winnipeg, eight cyclists were found to have amphetamine-related compounds in their urine. During the same year, several cyclists failed doping tests at the World Championships in Amsterdam. Five were found to be using amphetamines, six using ephedrine and two had been taking strychnine.

Many governing bodies had refused to accept that doping ever took place in their sport. Within those organisations that acknowledged the problem, officials believed that the introduction of dope testing would discourage the use of drugs. However, a tragic event in 1967 shattered this illusion, and also threatened to wreck the sport of professional cycling. Tommy Simpson, an ex-world professional road-racing champion, died whilst cycling in the most prestigious cycling event of all, the Tour de France. Simpson was only 29 and the cause of death was attributed to heart failure caused by heat exhaustion, lack of oxygen, humidity and overwork. However, it was not revealed until weeks later that traces of amphetamine, methylamphetamine (both stimulant drugs) and cognac were found in his body. Traces of amphetamine were also found in Simpson's jersey pockets, and drugs were found in his luggage. There was nothing new about a doping-related death but the impact of Tommy Simpson's death was enormous. This was mainly due to the prestige of the event and to the fact that this was the first doping death to be televised.

In the year following Simpson's death, the IOC set up a Medical Commission and introduced anti-doping legislation. They stated that any Olympic competitor 'who refuses to take a doping test or who is found guilty of doping shall be eliminated. If the Olympic competitor belongs to a team, the match or competition in question shall be forfeited by the team.' Furthermore, 'a medal may be withdrawn by order of the Executive Board on a proposal of the Medical Commission'. In 1968 random doping tests were carried out at the Winter Olympics in Grenoble and the Summer Olympics in Mexico City for *all* competitions. Testing was carried out for various types of stimulants, painkillers, anti-depressants and the 'major' tranquillisers. In certain competitions alcohol was often used to reduce tension but following the case of an intoxicated marksman at the Tokyo Olympics, excess alcohol was also banned in shooting and fencing competitions. All 86 of the drug tests at Grenoble, and 667 of the 668 tests at Mexico City, were negative. The exception was Hans-Gunnar Liljenvall who had a blood alcohol level above the limit of 40mg/100ml during the biathlon contest. As a result Liljenvall and his team mate Hans Jacobson lost the bronze medal, despite his plea that he had only drunk a couple of beers.

Doping-related incidents became more commonplace and sensational. In March 1968 the British runner Alan Simpson revealed to the media that he had taken amphetamines during the 1966 Commonwealth Games in Jamaica, at which he had won a silver medal. In the following August the Belgian distance runner Joseph Rombaux was disqualified for a positive dope test after winning the national marathon championship. He was banned from athletics for life. During the same year, there were two more doping-related deaths, both in Grenoble, France. Amphetamines were held to be responsible for the deaths of the soccer player Jean-Louis Quadri and the cyclist

Yves Mottin. In 1969 the brilliant cyclist Eddy Merckx was disqualified from the Giro d'Italia after failing a dope test. However, the suspension was lifted when it was revealed that a spectator had doped a drink and given it to Merckx. Eight competitors in the 1970 World weightlifting championships were disqualified for taking amphetamines. Over the next 2 years the Dutchman, de Noorlander, and four West German athletes, Heinfried Birlenbach, Erich Klamma, Renhard Kuretzky and Hermann Latzel were all suspended for using illegal substances in various events.

At the 1972 Games in Munich over 2000 urine samples were tested for drugs. Nine positive results were obtained and seven athletes were subsequently disqualified, including four medallists. The drugs detected were the stimulants ephedrine (3), nikethamide (2), phenmetrazine (1) and amphetamine (1). The results showed one of the main effects of the anti-doping regulations: enterprising athletes were turing to a much wider range of drugs in the hope of avoiding detection.

The most publicised case in Munich was that of the American swimmer, Rick DeMont, who had just won a gold medal in the 400m freestyle. After the event, ephedrine was detected in his urine; as a result he lost his medal and was disqualified from the remaining events. DeMont was unfortunate in that an anti-asthmatic drug he had been taking contained traces of ephedrine. Prior to competing, DeMont had reported the drug (Marex) on his medical records to officials, yet he was still disqualified. To many observers, the penalty imposed on DeMont appeared rather severe. There was such controversy over the issue that the IOC agreed to permit certain types of anti-asthmatic drugs at future Games. Prior to the 1976 Olympics, 51 members of the American team were questioned about their medications. *Sixteen* were unknowingly using banned drugs, and substitute drugs were found.

Alois Schloder, the captain of the West German ice-hockey team, was disqualified at the Winter Games in Sapporo, Japan, after failing a dope test. The atmosphere of the Games had already been soured by the disqualifications of the Austrian skier, Karl Schranz, and the French skier, Annie Famose.

While stimulants were being used to increase physical endurance in some sports, the tension of others was being reduced with anti-anxiety drugs. There were strong allegations from Major Monty Mortimer, manager of the British modern pentathlon team, that certain East European athletes were using sophisticated relaxant drugs. The protests followed the fall of Britain's Jim Fox from first to fifth position after the shooting events. Although the East Europeans did not fail the doping tests, Major Mortimer commented 'I don't believe that young athletes can shoot like this unless they have had a needle of some sort.' No evidence of excess alcohol was obtained in the 56 samples from contestants in the shooting events of modern pentathlon, but three did contain diazepam (Valium) and *ten* samples contained chlordiazepoxide (Librium). These anti-anxiety drugs or minor tranquillisers were not on the banned list, but were clearly being used instead of alcohol to 'steady nerves' during the competitions. Further developments during 1972 included the removal of the major tranquillisers from the banned list, because many doctors were prescribing them to athletes suffering from jet-lag. Local anaesthetic injections were also approved provided advance notice was given to the IOC Medical Committee.

In the 1974 European championships, the Russian athlete Vladimir Zhaloshik was positively dope-tested and disqualified after winning a bronze medal in the 20km walk. The Canadian middle-distance runner Joan Wenzel was also disqualified from third place at the 1975 Pan-American Games after traces of amphetamine were detected. She was banned for life, but was reinstated on appeal a year later. The International Amateur Athletics Federation (IAAF) accepted her explanation that she unwittingly took a cold treatment containing the drug. Unlike DeMont, she failed to declare it prior to the competition. Although it was not considered to be 'a case of drug-taking to improve performance', Wenzel was not allowed to keep her bronze medal.

The Russian cross-country skier Galina Kulakova failed a dope test after winning a bronze medal at the 1976 Winter Olympics in Innsbruck. Kulakova, who had won three gold medals at Sapporo, had used a nasal spray to relieve the symptoms of a heavy cold. She was disqualified when traces of ephedrine were detected. Her medal was handed over to another Russian, Nina Baldicheva, but the IOC allowed her to compete in the remaining events in Innsbruck.

Many sporting bodies now felt that the doping problem was firmly under control. They thought the pressures of international competition had caused the use of drugs in certain sports, but with routine, random testing, the problem was quietly and efficiently being removed from sport. In view of the harsh penalties associated with detection, it was not surprising that many officials shared this opinion. However, many athletes still used drugs which were either not on the banned list or were not detectable at the time. This was particularly true for the most widely publicised drugs, the anabolic steroids.

The use of anabolic steroids to increase body weight had been steadily increasing through the 1960s. They were used by body-builders in America during the late 1950s and then later by athletes in the 'heavy' events such as weightlifting, hammer-throwing and the shot-put. There were no rules against steroid use at this time and the techniques required to detect them were not available. However, it was becoming obvious to athletes, doctors and officials that competitors in certain events were becoming abnormally large. According to Olympic records the average weight of shot-putters increased by 14 per cent between 1956 and 1972. Despite several protests, anabolic steroids were not included on the IOC list of banned substances in 1968. At the time, no-one was aware of the long-term effects of steroids on health or whether they actually *did* improve performance. Yet many athletes continued to use steroids (in very large doses) as part of their training programme, simply because they appeared to promote muscle development.

Anabolic steroids were banned by the IAAF and the US Amateur Athletic Union in 1970 and 1971, but their use was already widespread by this time. In Munich the world record holder in the discus, Jay Silvester of the USA, conducted a survey among fellow athletes from seven nations. He found that *two-thirds* of competitors had taken steroids at least some time during their training periods. Some *61 per cent* had used them during the 6 months prior to the Games. With the exception of long-distance running, their use was prevalent among most track and field events. Harold Connolly, the American athlete, revealed that for 8 years prior to 1972 he was using anabolic steroids as an integral part of his training. Connolly claimed that in the American team of 1968 there were athletes with so many puncture holes from injected drugs that it was difficult to find a fresh injection site. Jeff Teale, a British Olympic shot-put finalist in 1968 and Commonwealth silver medallist in 1970, also admitted in an interview that he took steroids. He started on a quarter of a tablet per day in 1967 and by the end of 1972 was taking *ten* tablets per day. Teale was declared ineligible for international competition by the British Amateur Athletic Board, following his public admission and his failure to discuss the matter with them.

In January 1974 a new system of steroid testing was carried out at the Commonwealth Games in Christchurch, New Zealand. This followed a major breakthrough in detection methods by a research group led by Professor Brooks at St. Thomas's Hospital, London[6]. They developed a very sensitive test for screening blood and urine samples based on a technique known as radioimmunoassay. Random tests showed nine positive samples out of 55 competitors who were selected at the Games. However, the names or the sports of the guilty competitors were never revealed.

Once the detection methods were available, the IOC Medical Commission added anabolic steroids to their banned list and recommended testing at subsequent Olympic Games. The IAAF also announced that anyone found to have used steroids from January 1st 1975 would be banned from competitions. At the 1975 European Cup Finals the Bulgarian discus thrower Velko Velev and the Romanian shot-putter Valentina Cioltan were the first athletes to be found guilty of taking anabolic steroids. By the time of the 1976 Winter Games in Innsbruck, Austria, the IOC anti-doping legislation had become extremely complex. There were lists of *types* of banned drugs, specifically banned drugs, specifically permitted drugs and various regulations regarding nose drops, painkillers and anti-asthma preparations.

Testing for anabolic steroids was carried out at the 1976 Montreal Games by Robert Dugal and Michel Bertrand from the University of Quebec. They coupled radioimmunoassay procedures with other expensive but highly accurate techniques. As in the previous Olympics, over 2000 samples were tested, including 283 for steroids. There were 11 positive tests, eight of which were positive for steroids. All but one of the guilty competitors were weightlifters, the exception being Danuta Rosani of Poland[7]. Rosani did not compete in the discus final after failing the steroid test following the qualifying competition. Therefore she became the first athlete to be disqualified for using steroids in the Olympic arena. The disqualification also emphasised that *female* athletes were now using anabolic steroids.

Once appropriate testing procedures had been developed, the number of disqualifications soared. The following examples are only *some* of the most publicised cases. At the 1977 European Finals in Helsinki three Finnish athletes, Seppo Hovinen, Asko Pesonen and Markku Tuokko; one Russian, Vera Zapkaleno; and the East German, Ilona Slupianek, were all disqualified following positive tests. Slupianek was banned for a year, during which she was able to train presumably without the risk of being tested. Sixteen days after completing the ban, Slupianek won the European women's shot put in Prague with a championship record. Again there were cries of protest. While the 12 month suspensions were supposed to be acting as deterrents, they were regarded by many as potentially counter-productive, since they allowed the guilty athletes 12 test-free months. The result sparked off a new controversy which was only partly resolved when, later in the year, the IAAF voted to increase the *minimum* ban for a first positive dope test from 12 to 18 months.

The Norwegian, Knut Hjeltnes, and Walter Schmidt of Germany were also banned for using drugs during 1977; Barry Williams of Great Britain was also banned after newspaper allegations of drug use. Williams was reinstated in 1978. More disqualifications followed at the 1978 European Games. These included the Bulgarian, Elena Stoyanova, the Russians Yevgeniy Mironov, Vasiliy Yershov, Yekaterina Gordiyenko and the pentathlon gold medallist, Nadyezhda Tkachenko. However, it was not just athletes from Eastern bloc countries who were using steroids. During the same year the West German team champions, Hans-Joachim Krug (shot put) and Hein-Direck Neu (discus) were both banned. Two other discus throwers, the American Dave Voorhees and Briton, Colin Sutherland, were both banned from international competition after refusing to take a dope test.

Two Russian discus throwers, Yelena Kovalyeva and Nadya Kudryavtseva, were disqualified after positive tests at the 1979 European Junior Games, while at the 1979 Balkan Games five athletes were banned for taking anabolic steroids. These included the Bulgarian hurdler, Daniela Teneva, and the Romanian long-jumper, Sanda Vlad. However, the remaining athletes were three of the fastest female 1500m runners in the world. They were Totka Petrova, the World Cup winner, Natalia Marasescu of Romania, the former world mile record holder and Ileana Silai of Romania, the 1968 Olympic silver medallist. This suggested that top *middle-distance* runners were using steroids, and was also significant in that even if the athletes were reinstated after the statutory 18 month ban, they would miss the 1980 Moscow Olympics. The five athletes appealed to the Council of the IAAF for clemency. The controversy was heightened when the IAAF decided to reinstate the athletes from July 1st 1980, in time for the Olympics and with 11 'test-free' months in which to train. The Council was split 8 votes to 8, and the motion was carried by the casting vote of the President, Adriaan Paulen[8].

14

There were protests at the reinstatement from around the world, and the IAAF Council member Arne Llungqvist publicly dissociated himself from the decision. The British athlete Christine Benning conducted a personal boycott of the Games in protest at the reinstatement while Mary Purcell from the Irish Republic also refused to go to Moscow. Adriaan Paulen attempted to defuse the situation by admitting 'surprise' at the weight of opinion against his decision. He eventually admitted that the decision was wrong and urged an even tougher clampdown on doping in the future. None of the 'prematurely' reinstated athletes won medals at Moscow. Silai and Marasescu finished eighth and ninth respectively in the women's 1500m final, while Petrova failed in her heat. However, there were still protests concerning other athletes who had completed bans for doping, who were now able to compete in the Games. In particular, Slupianek and Tkachenko, who had both completed their 18-month suspensions, won gold medals in the shot put and pentathlon respectively at Moscow. The disqualifications and the associated arguments continued at several subsequent athletic meetings.

At the 1980 Winter Olympics at Lake Placid, USA, there were no positive tests. One triumphant bobsleigh team almost lost a medal when they reported late to the sample station after having been delayed by television interviewers. In April 1980 Ronald Desruelles was disqualified for drug use after winning the long jump at the European Indoor Championships in West Germany. The following year the shot-putter Nonu Abashdze of the Soviet Union and Karoline Kafer, an Austrian sprinter, were both banned after positive tests at the Indoor Games. At the 1981 Pacific Conference Games Gael Mulhall of Australia, and the American Ben Plucknett, both winners in the discus, were disqualified after failing dope tests.

The 1983 Pan-American Games in Caracas, Venezuela, were obviously regarded by some athletes as a fairly 'relaxed' occasion in terms of dope testing. However they were proved wrong in their assumption and *eleven* weightlifters from nine countries were found to have taken steroids. Thirteen American competitors (all track and field athletes) immediately packed their bags and went home before competing.

The organisers of the 1984 Olympic Games in Los Angeles spent over 1.6 *million* dollars to establish sophisticated doping controls, and the disqualifications soon followed. Two Canadian weightlifters, Terry Hadlow and Luc Chagnon, were sent home before competing, when samples taken during training periods prior to the Games proved positive. During competition the weightlifters Mahmoud Tahra of Lebanon and Ahmed Tarbi of Algeria were both banned for life from international competition following positive tests.

Martti Vainio of Finland became the first medal-winning athlete to be disqualified from the Games for taking drugs. Vainio finished second in the 10,000m but lost the silver medal which was handed over to Britain's Mike McLeod. Vainio was also banned from the 5000m final. The disqualification surprised many observers. As Carl-Olaf Homen, vice chairman of the Finnish delegation said, 'Vainio is the last person I would have expected it of. The 33-year-old former European champion protested his innocence and said he had not knowingly taken any steroids. He wanted new tests in Finland on the 'vitamins' he had taken, to determine whether any contained steroids. After arriving in Helsinki, he said 'I have to carry the burden. My career as a sportsman is apparently over.'

In November 1984 it was revealed that *prior* to the Olympic Games, Vainio had already been found guilty of doping. A positive test had been reported at the 1984 Rotterdam marathon in April. The result was hushed up, presumably because it would have prevented Vainio representing Finland in Los Angeles. The chief national coach Antti Lanamaki resigned after admitting responsibility for the cover-up. The national distance running coach Timo Vuorimaa was also severely reprimanded by the Finnish Athletic Association for his involvement.

Following her disqualification in Los Angeles, Anna Verouli, Greece's European javelin champion, who was also found to have taken steroids, said she wanted a second test. The Swedish wrestler Thomas Johansson was also stripped of his silver medal following a positive dope test. These disqualifications demonstrate that while the popular Press regards drug use as part of the State-controlled sports training programme of the Eastern bloc, doping is also prevalent among Western athletes.

Although the methods used to detect steroids have *possibly* reduced the incidence of anabolic steroid use, many athletes are still taking drugs of some kind to improve performance. There is now increasing evidence that athletes are using substances which are not yet on the banned list, or using substances such as testosterone, which are already found in the body and hence bans are more difficult to enforce[9]. Re-tests on urine samples at both the 1980 Olympic Games in Lake Placid and Moscow revealed significant levels of testosterone. Athletes may also discontinue their use in enough time prior to the event to escape detection. While doping in sport is not new, what constitutes doping has changed dramatically, particularly over the last three decades. Perhaps more worrying is that doping appears to be firmly entrenched in many sports. Indeed, in some sports it has been suggested that it may be impossible to 'get to the top' without the use of these illegal substances.

The implication of the present chapter would appear to be that doping assures medals, yet this is *not* the case. The 'beneficial' effects of the drugs, widely accepted by athletes, are not always supported by the findings of controlled scientific studies. Moreover, many losing competitors have often used the same drugs as the winners. Are these benefits fact or fiction? The following chapters examine the question of whether these drugs do improve performance, their side effects and their long-term effects on health.

2
STIMULANTS

It's amazing the way Americans buy good tickets to watch speed freaks try to kill each other!
Dr. Arnold J. Mandell, referring to American football players, 1976.

The benefits athletes usually expect from 'stimulant' drugs include an increase in alertness and exercise endurance combined with a delay in the onset of fatigue. Therefore, many individuals have used stimulant drugs in sports where physical fitness is critical. As Chapter 1 revealed, stimulants have been popular in several sports, particularly in cycling and soccer, sometimes with *fatal* consequences. Certain stimulants are also known to affect behaviour by producing 'rage' responses which has prompted their use in sports such as American football where extra 'aggression' is required/Most people are aware that the use of stimulant drugs such as amphetamines is illegal in many countries, yet the use of other stimulants such as caffeine (found in drinks such as coffee) obviously is not. These drugs produce their effects in different ways, but it is necessary to examine some basic physiology to understand these differences (see Appendix A).

During times of stress, the sympathetic nervous system is activated and noradrenalin, adrenalin and corticosteroids are released resulting in increased cardiac output, increased blood flow to the muscles and elevated blood sugar levels. These effects are clearly useful during exercise since they ensure that the muscles receive a constant supply of oxygen and nutrients and a rapid removal of potentially toxic waste products. Thus it is not surprising that drugs which mimic the effects of sympathetic stimulation have been used by athletes to improve performance. These are called the 'sympathomimetic amines'. However, their use by athletes is banned by the IOC as shown in Table 2.1.

TABLE 2.1   Examples of sympathomimetic amines currently banned by the IOC

Chlorprenaline	Isoprenaline
Ephedrine	Methoxyphenamine
Etafedrine	Methylephedrine
Isoetharine	and related compounds

It is interesting that ephedrine is on the banned list. This was the substance detected in the anti-asthma preparation used by Rick DeMont (see Chapter 1). Ephedrine dilates the bronchi or tiny air sacs in the lungs which brings some relief to asthma patients. This presented a problem for a choice of permitted medication in the treatment of asthma and respiratory ailments. At present, other *selective* stimulants called beta-agonists are used to treat asthma (e.g. salbutamol and terbutaline)[1]. Some of the drugs can only be administered to athletes on condition that the IOC Medical Commission gives its agreement following a report of the team doctor.

Many medications which act as nasal decongestants also contain at least some sympathomimetic amines as their active ingredients. In June of 1984 the British-Canadian Ronald Angus made legal history in Britain when he appealed against a life-time ban for drug-taking. It was believed to be the first time any sportsman had challenged a governing body's decision on drugs in a British court[2]. Angus won the all-England judo championship in December of 1983 and was banned 11 days later after allegations of drug-taking. He had been taking a drug

19

with the trade name Sudafed which had been prescribed by his Canadian doctor. He claimed that it was prescribed as a nasal decongestant, that he was told it was not banned and that it would not affect performance. However, the preparation actually contained an ephedrine-like substance which was banned.

Angus was reinstated after the British Judo Association admitted that the life ban and 5-year suspension from membership was 'against the rules of natural justice'. The reinstatement was in time to enable Angus to participate in trials for the Los Angeles Olympics, but the case illustrated the problems of permitting nasal decongestants. Since the derivatives of the substance imidazoline have no stimulant effects on the central nervous system, they *are* permitted as decongestants. Examples of these drugs include nafazoline (Privine), tetrahydrozoline (Tyzine) and xylometazoline (Otrivine).

There is actually little evidence that the drugs listed in Table 2.1 improve athletic performance. Indeed, while the amines are useful for their anti-asthmatic or decongestant properties, it is unlikely that the amounts found in these preparations would significantly affect performance. However, ephedrine *can* increase blood pressure by directly increasing cardiac output and causing the release of noradrenalin from sympathetic nerve endings. At higher doses ephedrine can act on the brain, causing nausea and dizziness, and if taken at night may prevent sleep. Thus while these drugs could *potentially* improve some aspects of performance, there are important side effects to be considered. With sympathomimetic amines it would seem reasonable to test for *how* much of the substance was in the body, in order to distinguish between those who are taking the drug for its therapeutic benefits and those are using it as a doping agent.

A hormone from the adrenal glands, adrenalin, is released during times of fear or stress. Injections of adrenalin increase heart rate and blood pressure and may raise the level of blood glucose. These effects could potentially improve athletic performance. However, there is little scientific evidence to suggest that adrenalin injections are beneficial in endurance tests[3]. The number of athletes who have been disqualified for using sympathomimetic amines is fairly small, which contrasts sharply with the number of disqualifications for abuse of the so–called 'psychomotor stimulant' drugs.

The psychomotor stimulants are mainly synthetic drugs, although some, such as cocaine, do occur naturally. Cocaine is found in coca leaves which were chewed by South American natives to help them to walk or toil for prolonged periods without experiencing tiredness. By contrast, amphetamine was produced in 1887 and its derivative benzedrine was synthesised in America in 1934. Since then, there have been a range of amphetamine-like products developed and only some are shown in Table 2.2. Their slang names include 'bennies', 'dexys', 'greenies', 'pep-pills' or more commonly 'speed'.

TABLE 2.2   Examples of psychomotor stimulant drugs currently banned by the IOC

Amphetamine	Norpseudoephedrine
Benzphetamine	Pemoline
Chlorphentamine	Phencanphamine
Cocaine	Phendimetrazine
Diethylpropion	Phentermine
Dimethylamphetamine	Pipradol
Ethylmphetamine	Preolintane
Meclofenoxate	and related compounds
Methylamphetamine	
Methylfenidate	

The effects of psychomotor stimulants are similar to the sympathomimetic amines in that they increase heart rate, respiration and blood pressure and generally enhance the activity of the sympathetic nervous system. However, they also have a stimulant action on the *brain*. Someone taking these stimulants feels alert, light-headed or even euphoric. The drugs promote a powerful feeling of well-being and confidence. To understand how these drugs produce these effects, it is necessary to examine briefly the physiology of the central nervous system.

The brain is composed of thousands of millions of nerve cells or neurons. It is known that 'messages' are passed along neurons by means of electrical impulses, and that a chemical called a 'neurotransmitter' carries the information from one neuron to another. Each cell may receive messages from thousands of other cells and may then pass information to thousands of other cells, thus the whole picture is very complex. It is now known that pathways in the brain use particular chemicals as their transmitter substance and it has also been possible to identify several of these substances. There is evidence that noradrenalin and dopamine are neurotransmitters, and their roles seem particularly linked with the control of certain aspects of behaviour and mood. What is relevant to the present discussion is that drugs which affect behaviour or mood may do so by affecting the activity of neurotransmitters in these brain pathways. A whole range of drugs have been developed to either increase or decrease the activity of these transmitters. This has provided neuroscientists with a greater understanding of how the brain controls various aspects of behaviour, and has provided insight into some forms of mental illness.

One of the effects of amphetamine is to *increase* the production and release of dopamine and noradrenalin in parts of the brain known as the limbic system. Amphetamine stimulates areas that activate 'arousal' and 'reward' mechanisms. Thus amphetamine can increase arousal and elevate mood by acting on the brain. It also increases the release of neurotransmitters in that part of the brain which initiates movement, so increasing motor activity. In view of its psychological and physiological effects, the use of amphetamines appears to be potentially beneficial, but does it improve athletic performance?

In terms of endurance, amphetamines can *prolong* performance. Soldiers forced to march long distances and given amphetamines were willing to continue marching despite severe foot blisters. Football players taking amphetamines have been reported to play on despite pain from injury. In laboratory studies, amphetamines have also been shown to increase treadmill endurance times, using both human and animal subjects[4].

The most quoted studies regarding the effects of amphetamines on athletic performance were published over 20 years ago by Gene Smith and Henry Beecher[5]. They tested athletes on three classes of performance: swimming, running and weight throwing either following a control treatment or treatment with amphetamine. This was a 'double-blind' study in which neither the experimenters nor the athletes knew which treatment was being administered at the time. Fourteen out of fifteen swimmers improved with amphetamine treatment, although the improvements were small, usually in the order of +1 per cent. In the running events the results were more varied, but again amphetamines tended to improve performance. Nineteen out of 26 runners were faster following amphetamine treatment.

Thus the results supported laboratory findings in that the drug appeared to delay the onset of fatigue and improve performance. Smith and Beecher also reported that the drug improved performance when a brief, explosive response was needed. For example, the shot-putters and weight throwers also improved the average distance of their throws with amphetamine.

The differences were again fairly small, usually in the region of +4 per cent. They concluded that amphetamine made the athletes *feel* more vigorous, alert and energetic and suggested that amphetamines could enhance both short-term and prolonged performance.

However, there are several problems with the studies conducted by Smith and Beecher. For example, they used a small dose range of amphetamine, they used a range of distances for running events varying from 600 yards to 12 miles, in which the athletes were sometimes allowed to time themselves, and they compared results across different weather conditions. Furthermore, there have been several large studies which have been more carefully controlled that have not found beneficial effects after amphetamine treatment[6]. A more recent study was carried out by Joe Chandler and Steven Blair at the University of South Carolina in 1980[7]. Treatment with Dexedrine improved performance in terms of knee extension strength, acceleration, and time to exhaustion. Even though the time to exhaustion was increased, there was no difference in sprinting speed. Any effects observed were typically very small. There have been several other studies which have either reported 'mixed' benefits or very small effects[8].

The size of changes in performance induced by amphetamine may be tiny, even as little as 1 per cent[9]. Nevertheless, this 1 per cent improvement can make the difference between 'fame and oblivion'. Victor Laties and Bernard Weiss use the world record times for the mile as an example. Over the last hundred years, there has only been a 15 per cent improvement. On average, it takes about 7 years for a 1 per cent improvement. Thus if a drug can improve performance by 1 per cent an athlete will suddenly be years ahead of his or her time. Laties and Weiss suggest that there is an 'amphetamine margin' and conclude that amphetamine is called 'speed' for good reason.

However, there is *still* a need for carefully controlled studies using a range of doses and sports before any definitive statements could be made. Even then, there are still limitations. The competing athlete may be using doses *far* in excess of those permitted in laboratory studies. Furthermore, the tests do not reproduce the conditions associated with the pressures, atmosphere and stress of the actual event. Nevertheless, if we tentatively accept that amphetamines can produce small *but* crucial improvements in some aspects of performance, why don't more athletes use them?

The truth is that there are many adverse reactions to these psychomotor stimulants, particularly when higher doses are taken. There are several cardiovascular reactions such as heart palpitations and high blood pressure. The latter can lead to severe headaches or even brain haemorrhages. There are also gastrointestinal side effects such as constipation or diarrhoea. There may also be various hormonal reactions resulting in loss of libido and impotence. If that were not enough, these drugs also are highly addictive. For example, amphetamines were given to Japanese servicemen during the Second World War. In less than 10 years, the number of known addicts had risen from a few to over 200,000!

Amphetamines are often abused because of the psychological 'high' they can produce. However, the body develops a rapid tolerance to the drug and the user needs an increasing dose to obtain the excitatory or euphoric effects. Withdrawal from the drug produces periods of severe depression. Thus, once an athlete becomes 'hooked' on these stimulants, he or she may be unable to perform without them and eventually perform only with very high doses. Since most drugs are toxic if taken in very high doses, there is also the possibility of an overdose.

There are also several psychological and behavioural reactions that can interfere with the athlete's performance. In addition to headaches, the athlete may become restless, agitated or have difficulty getting to sleep. This may lead to cases of impaired judgement and the periods of amphetamine-induced euphoria may alternate with periods of apathy and depression. Finally, large doses of amphetamine produce symptoms almost identical to those seen in patients with paranoid schizophrenia! Indeed, there have been individuals who have been diagnosed as paranoid schizophrenic who were later found to have taken an enormous dose of amphetamine. These 'amphetamine psychoses' are characterised by hallucinations (where the person 'hears' voices or 'sees' things) and feelings of persecution, whereby the person feels everyone is 'out to get him'. As a result, the person behaves very irrationally or *aggressively*. The symptoms of amphetamine psychosis eventually disappear, once the person 'dries out' and discontinues drug-use. Despite these potential risks, athletes continue to use amphetamines and other stimulant drugs.

Amphetamines have been used by rally-drivers seeking extra endurance. While this may ensure that the driver stays awake and *apparently* alert, the drug may produce impaired judgement. Rumours have abounded of students in examinations who wrote gibberish or simply kept writing their name over and over again after taking amphetamines. Certainly, repetitive or 'stereotyped' behaviour is a characteristic feature of amphetamine intoxication. Many of these drugs also have anorectic properties, i.e. they reduce appetite and cause weight loss, and have been used clinically to treat some forms of obesity. Amphetamines and related compounds have been used by jockeys and boxers to get down to the appropriate weight for their sport. The loss of appetite produced by the drug is probably as a result of the main effects that have been described. Owing to the potential risks, they should only be used under careful medical supervision for this purpose.

Chapter 1 illustrated how there was an 'amphetamine era' in the recent history of doping with *fatal* consequences. Many of these athletes died at the peak of their fitness because the drugs removed or made the user unaware of the physiological signals which act to prevent over exertion. For example, the effects of amphetamine include shunting blood from the skin to the muscles which limits the natural cooling effect of the body. In the intense heat in Rome, Jensen died of what appeared to be sunstroke, because his body was unable to cool itself after amphetamine treatment. Similarly, Simpson died of heart failure caused by heat exhaustion. Due to the psychological effects of the drug, neither cyclist was able to recognise this point of exhaustion, and continued cycling to the point of 'blacking out'. Other cyclists have actually been lucky to collapse before reaching this point.

The long-term effects and dangers of amphetamine use were not fully recognised during the 1950s or early 1960s. Despite the risks that emerged, many athletes were still prepared to 'take the chance' or 'experiment' in the hope of achieving the 'amphetamine margin'. As testing methods have improved, stimulant use has declined, yet we still hear of athletes from a variety of sports who are disqualified for stimulant use. In the 1981 European Cup semi-finals the Hungarian shot-putter Laszlo Szabo and the Austrian hurdler Evelyn Ledl were both banned for stimulant use. Other offenders have included weightlifters, runners, cyclists and soccer players.

In the 1978 World Cup in Argentina, the Scottish soccer player Willie Johnston was found to have taken the stimulant drug phencamphamine before Scotland's game with Peru[10]. Johnston was the second player in World Cup history to be banned for dope-taking, the first being Ernst Jean-Joseph of Haiti in 1974. Had the event been an Olympic competition, the whole team would probably been disqualified; however only Johnston was sent home. The whole episode raised several questions, particularly about professional players using stimulant drugs on a regular basis at club level. Certainly, soccer at this level fitted the description of a sport especially prone to doping. Matches are frequently over a long season, the rewards are directly related to success and the amount of money involved is high. Most soccer careers are relatively short so the pressures to succeed early are intense.

Many observers, including Professor Arnold Beckett, a leading campaigner against the use of drugs in sport, had long spoken of the 'smug attitude' of British soccer towards doping, despite a number of rumours and 'revelations' to the popular press[11]. Certainly the authorities were relatively slow to take the appropriate measures. Following the Johnston episode and the press outcry, the Football Association (FA) conducted an inquiry in late 1979 but found no evidence of drug-taking among soccer players in England. One hundred and fifty-five players were tested for stimulant use. Currently, the FA conducts a limited programme of testing during the season, incorporating both Football League and FA Cup-ties[12]. The testing and analysis of samples are carried out by Professor Beckett's research team at the Chelsea College Drug Testing Centre in London. A programme of tests is constructed at the start of the season to cover a range of clubs from each League Division and *two* players are randomly selected from each team at each match covered. Clubs are obviously not informed that a test will be conducted at their ground until the testers present themselves during the second half of a match.

Doping tests were not introduced into European soccer competitions until 1980. The list of prohibited drugs used by the International and European Football Associations (FIFA and EUFA) are similar to that used by the IOC. So far, there have

27

been no reported cases of doping in European matches. In sharp contrast, American football seems to have been a fertile ground for the use of drugs and in particular, the psychomotor stimulants[13].

The use of amphetamines in American football was officially banned by the National Football League (NFL) in 1971. The NFL acted when several players sued and won large financial settlements for drug-related injuries in San Diego, St. Louis, Chicago and Toronto (the last was not a NFL city, but had a team with ex–NFL players). The extent of amphetamine use in either the Canadian or American leagues was obviously difficult to assess, but the problem was publicised by a number of retired players and by an eminent psychiatrist, Arnold J. Mandell.

Mandell was 'caught' giving amphetamines to members of the San Diego Chargers team. Some of the players referred to Mandell as 'the benny boy' (i.e. the person who brought the bennies or amphetamines), and he was dismissed in 1974 after the NFL accused him of giving out 1750 amphetamine pills (5 to 15 mg each) over a 3-month period. Two players were reported to have received 400 pills each. Two years later Mandell published a sensational account of his experiences in a book entitled *The Nightmare Season* [14]. In 1978 he was reprimanded by the California Board of Medical Quality Assurance for writing 'clearly excessive' amphetamine prescriptions for the team. He later appealed against the medical board decision to the state superior court. Mandell insisted that he was being used as a scapegoat for speaking out on a subject the NFL preferred not to hear about. Arnold Mandell was the founding chairman of the Department of Psychiatry at San Diego, is a recognised expert on neurochemistry, is the recipient of millions of dollars in research grants, and is the author of several books and hundreds of scientific papers. Consequently, many people were prepared to listen to what he had to say on the subject.

Mandell continued to be a thorn in the NFL's side by providing more information on the use of amphetamines in professional football. He tabulated the quantities of drugs used by the Chargers in 1968 and 1969, and conducted interviews with several players (see Table 2.3). In September 1978 he presented the data in a paper called 'The Sunday Syndrome' at a national conference on amphetamine held in San Francisco[15]. The results came as a severe shock to many people involved in American football. He reported that players typically used amphetamines once a week, during the game on Sunday. Using the drugs this way, the effects were more powerful than if the players took them daily. Their use was particularly prevalent among older players and those playing in defensive positions. What was most stunning was the dose ranges involved. Mandell estimated that the average dose was between 60 and 70mg per player per game, and the highest dose was *150mg per game*. These doses are extremely high and would certainly produce the hostility, paranoia and aggression characteristic of the 'amphetamine rage' reaction. Given the level of violence in the sport, the extra 'aggression' might well *appear* to be useful. Players who were aware of the risks may have decided that the benefits outweighed them. Furthermore, if players thought that members of the opposition team were using amphetamines, they may be tempted to match them drug for drug. Amphetamine also dulls feelings of pain, thus enabling the player to continue despite the bruises and abrasions characteristic of this type of 'contact' sport (see Table 2.4).

Mandell conceded that he wrote very large prescriptions, but claimed he was beginning to treat people with a long-term addiction. All of his 'patients' had been using amphetamines for at least 9 years. He argued that team trainers had routinely handed out envelopes of benzedrine and dexedrine before games. By writing prescriptions, he could protect players from turning to black market sources and win their co-operation in a programme of self-reform. The players generally regarded the drug as a 'work drug' rather than a drug for abuse.

The NFL had begun a drug control and monitoring system in 1975, whereby clubs sent copies of their medical supply order form to NFL headquarters and had also begun a major drug education programme. However, according to Mandell, this was not the answer to the problem. He argued that prohibition

TABLE 2.3   Incidence of amphetamine use by professional football
players interviewed

Position	Yes	No	Occasionally	Dose range (mg/Sunday)
Wide receiver	6	5	2	5–15
Quarterback	1	8	0	10–15
Defensive back	7	4	2	5–10
Running back	8	3	2	5–25
Tight end	2	2	1	10–30
Linebacker	5	4	1	10–60
Offensive lineman	10	4	0	15–105
Defensive lineman	9	0	1	30–150
Totals	48	30	9	5–150

Reproduced by permission[15].

TABLE 2.4   Dose ranges and expected effects of amphetamine
administration on American football players

Dose	NDL position	Rationale
5–10 mg	Quarterback Wide receiver Defensive back	Creative performance Energy
15–45 mg	Special team Linebacker Offensive linesman	Fearlessness Stability
50–200 mg	Defensive end Defensive tackle	Manic high Paranoid rage

Reproduced by permission[15].

would simply drive the problem 'underground' and players
would turn to black market sources. Although the San Diego
team was the only one disciplined, Mandell argued that the
pattern of abuse he described was 'normative and systematic' in
American professional football. He said the competitive advan-

tage given by amphetamines was 'enormous' and also suggested that amphetamines may be responsible for the increasing incidence of reported injuries in the game. He stated that the only way to wipe out amphetamine abuse would be to have urine tests for *all* players before *every game*. Mandell believes this will never happen because several popular football 'stars' would be disqualified and because the public *enjoy* the spectacle of violence in sport[16].

Most NFL officials do not accept Mandell's generalisations, based on his experience with the Chargers. They believe that there is only isolated use and regard mandatory urine testing as an invasion of the players' privacy. They suggest it could also be an 'unpleasant issue in contract negotiations' and neither the players nor the NFL desired the testing. Many players regard amphetamine use as passé, but have the players simply 'moved on' to other types of drugs? Until the NFL introduce doping tests, it will never be known.

One drug that is almost certainly abused by American football players is cocaine. Carl Eller, a defensive lineman for the Minnesota Vikings, estimated that as many as 40 per cent of all professional players are regular users of cocaine. This powerful stimulant can produce feelings of euphoria and is capable of improving some aspects of performance through prolonged endurance. However, larger doses produce muscle spasms and convulsions. Furthermore, cocaine increases body temperature which may contribute to heat illness. Since cocaine is reported to be a popular drug of abuse among wealthy 'stars', it has not surprising that it has been used by American football players. However, there have been some well-publicised casualities as a result. The ex-Miami Dolphin player 'Mercury' Morris recieved a 20-year prison sentence for selling cocaine, while Tony Peters of the Washington Redskins was arrested in August 1983 for cocaine-related offences. A few days later, four other players were fined and suspended for cocaine abuse. These were Greg Stemrick of the New Orleans Saints, E. J. Junior of the St. Louis Cardinals, Pete Johnson and Ross Browner, both of the Cincinnati Bengals. The baseball player,

31

Steve Howe of the Los Angeles Dodgers, was also fined after cocaine abuse[17].

The level of violence in other sports such as ice-hockey also arouses suspicion of possible stimulant abuse, but again reliable data are lacking. In his book *Ball Four*, Jim Bouton claims that 40 per cent of the major league baseball players in America used amphetamines, usually benzedrine[18]. He noted that players on amphetamines frequently feel that they are playing brilliantly, but their performance may be well below normal. Similarly, there have also been bicycle races where all participants were tested for amphetamines at the end of the race. Amphetamine traces were only found in those who had finished at the back of the pack[19]. Nevertheless, many cyclists still use stimulants.

Professional cyclists must endure a gruelling season racing day after day in country after country, and the temptation to use drugs is enormous. In 1984 the Irish cyclist Sean Kelly proved himself to be the world's top cyclist, winning a total of 32 races between March and October. But near the end of the season, Kelly failed a dope test after finishing third in the Paris to Brussels race[20]. Kelly protested his innocence and said that there had been irregularities in the testing. He suggested that there might have been a mix-up in the samples and said he was going to fight the 'injustice' in court with the backing of his sponsors. However, the second sample analysis was also positive. In October 1984 Kelly's appeal was rejected by the Belgian cycling federation for lack of firm evidence that the control had been conducted improperly. He was fined 1000 Swiss francs and received a 1-month ban suspended for a year. It was surprising to many observers that Kelly should use a drug. His successful season had led him to be tested 26 times and none were positive. If he did take the drug, he would have known he would be tested if he finished in the first four. The Belgian cycling authorities said his sample contained traces of 'Stimul', a stimulant rejected by most cyclists years ago as being unsophisticated. It was the first time in 8 years of racing and 8 years of doping controls that Kelly was found guilty.

The psychomotor stimulants *may* improve athletic performance in certain sports, probably as much through their psychological as their physical effects. In addition to the dangers of addiction, there are many adverse physical and psychological reactions which are detrimental to the users and even to fellow athletes through increased levels of aggression. These stimulants do not improve *skill*, but may increase endurance, so their benefits are limited. Amphetamines once had a place in medicine, for example treating asthma, low blood pressure and some forms of obesity, but they do not have a legitimate place in sport.

The final category of stimulants are simply referred to as 'miscellaneous central nervous stimulants' (see Table 2.5). Most

TABLE 2.5   Examples of miscellaneous stimulants currently banned by the IOC

Amiphenazole	Ethamivan
Bemigride	Leptazol
Caffeine	Nikethamide
Croproamide	Picrotoxin
Crotethamide	Strychnine
Doxapram	and related compounds

of the drugs in this category are extremely poisonous and should never be used without medical supervision. These drugs stimulate various parts of the central nervous system, but their most important actions are usually on part of the midbrain called the *medulla* which plays a vital role in the control of important functions such as respiration and heart rate (see Figure 2.1). These drugs are used clinically to overcome the effects of sleeping pill overdoses and are known as 'analeptic' drugs. Given in high doses they produce convulsions. For example, strychnine increases the reflex excitability of the spinal cord and the muscles respond in a co-ordinated manner. However, higher doses send all the voluntary muscles into violent and painful spasms and convulsions. After five or six convulsions, respiration fails to return and the recipient dies of asphyxiation. Due to their toxicity, these convulsants have not been

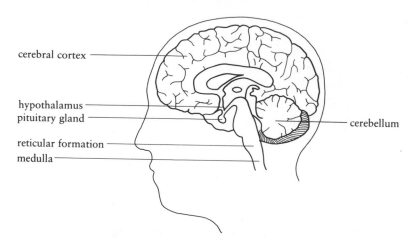

cerebral cortex

hypothalamus
pituitary gland

reticular formation
medulla

cerebellum

FIGURE 2.1   Section through the human brain showing some of the more important basic structures referred to in the text. The hypothalamus and pituitary form a link between the higher (intellectual) parts of the brain (e.g. the cerebral cortex) and the hormonal system. The cerebellum is partly responsible for the control of movement and balance while the medulla monitors the body's vegetative processes.

widely used as doping agents, although there are a few reported cases. Strychnine was supposedly used by the marathon runners Hicks and Pietri, and traces of the convulsant, nikethamide, were found in urine samples of two athletes at the Munich Games.

In contrast, caffeine has been used as a stimulant in several sports. Caffeine, which is found in coffee, tea, cocoa and cola, can produce 'clear' thought and reduce fatigue or drowsiness. It also improves 'higher' functions such as mental arithmetic. These effects can be obtained with about 100 to 250mg of caffeine, the amount contained in one or two cups of coffee. At recent Olympic Games, tests on urine samples revealed that some athletes had *very high* caffeine concentrations, which would have been impossible to achieve by drinking coffee. In these cases the caffeine was either taken orally as tablets, injected intramuscularly, or through the rectum by the use of suppositories[21].

Caffeine is a strong stimulant that excites the central nervous system at all levels, but particularly the cerebral cortex (see Figure 2.1). It is an effective respiratory stimulant by acting on the medulla, it increases heart rate, and acts as a diuretic, in other words, it increases the flow of urine. In excess, caffeine can produce insomnia, and if injected in large doses, produces strychnine-like convulsions by over-excitation of the spinal cord. Thus in reasonable doses caffeine can be a useful drug; in excess it is more dangerous.

In terms of respiratory, cardiac and muscle stimulation, caffeine could be regarded as a *potentially* useful substance for the athlete, but the effects are highly variable. There have been several controlled laboratory studies which have investigated the effects of caffeine on performance. In a 1978 study, cyclists exercised until exhaustion on an exercise bicycle after drinking either decaffeinated coffee or coffee containing 330mg of caffeine. The caffeine increased endurance time on the bicycle by 19 per cent! The following year, the same group conducted a similar study, and found that an injection of 250mg of caffeine increased work production by 7 per cent[22].

Caffeine is known to stimulate the mobilisation of free fatty acids and to increase the burn-up of fat. This is significant because although carbohydrates have generally been considered to be the primary, if not the only, fuel for muscular exercise, it is now recognised that the role of fat as a primary energy source during exercise is considerable. Since carbohydrate sources are limited, a substance which uses fat instead of carbohydrate would spare carbohydrate stores, and theoretically prolong exercise endurance. Therefore caffeine may increase endurance by increasing fat oxidation and sparing carbohydrates. However, several studies either do not report beneficial effects on performance following ingestion of caffeine, or report 'mixed' effects[23]. Thus, the 'benefits' reported have to be treated with some caution, since the effects seem to be highly variable. A regular user of caffeine may have developed a high tolerance level, and a beneficial effect may be difficult to demonstrate. The evidence suggesting that caffeine enhances performance is somewhat limited.

Because of the potentially harmful effects of caffeine, the Medical Commision of the IOC decided to ban *excess* caffeine. Urine samples were tested *quantitatively* at the 1984 Olympic Games at Sarajevo and Los Angeles. A specimen was considered positive if the concentration of caffeine in the urine exceeded 15 micrograms per ml (this is about ten times the level present after consuming an 'average' amount of coffee). No positive cases of caffeine doping have been reported and it remains to be seen whether other sports will also start testing for excess caffeine. Tea and coffee contain other stimulants such as theophylline and theobromine, although they are present only in very small quantities. Theophylline, which has many similar properties to caffeine, is permitted as an anti-asthmatic preparation. Theophylline's stimulant action on the brain is much weaker than that of caffeine. In higher doses it unfortunately produces gastric discomfort[24].

In general, the 'beneficial' effects of stimulants on athletic performance are questionable. Indeed, there are many risks associated with their use. Most types of stimulant drugs are now prohibited under present IOC Rules but there are still stimulant substances used by athletes which are not on the banned list. These will be discussed in Chapter 7 as part of the 'current trends' in doping, but one report is worth immediate attention. In the 1982 World Cup in Spain, the Italian soccer team had a dismal first round, but then underwent a dramatic recovery to beat the favourites Brazil, the defending champions Argentina, and West Germany in the final. The Italian press described the improvement as 'miraculous'. However, the Italian team doctor Leonardo Vecchiet hotly disputed reports that he gave the players a 'miracle treatment' to offset fatigue and help them to victory[25]. He admitted that he had given the players a product freely available in Spanish pharmacies which was 'not a drug'. A spokesman for the makers of this product, 'Carnitene' described it as 'a natural substance reproducing a muscle product that is recommended for heart patients and can cut down fatigue'. Dr. Vecchiet said that he had studied Carnitene for a year, and its usefulness was 'indisputable'. He told a Rome newspaper

> It was only one of a hundred things that allowed the back-up people to put the most efficient squad on the field. I find the moral that people are pretending to draw from this pretty dishonest.

Whether Carnitene reduces fatigue is debatable, but if the players *believed* it did, then it is significant. This so-called 'placebo' effect of treatments cannot be underestimated.

In the 1930s, 'monkey gland' extracts were given to soccer players to promote fitness. It is unlikely that these extracts of monkey (adrenal) gland would affect performance, for while they might contain substances such as noradrenalin, adrenalin or corticosteroids, they would be rapidly broken down in the body and excreted. What is important is that the players receiving the extracts *believed* they would increase endurance. Indeed, the young Wolverhampton Wanderers team soared to the top of the English First Division after apparently receiving monkey gland treatment. One popular account was that the team were so sure of their extra fitness that a wet ground gave them an advantage over their opponents. To ensure these conditions, they supposedly invited the local fire brigade to hose the pitch before home games[26]. Athletes are still buying 'animal gland' extracts (which are widely available) to enhance performance. As far as we are aware, there is *no* scientific evidence to suggest that these products improve any aspect of performance.

3

ANABOLIC STEROIDS

> . . . there is a substantial body of evidence that will stand very
> close scrutiny to indicate that anabolic steroids will not contri-
> bute significantly to gains in lean muscle bulk or muscle strength
> in healthy young adult males.
> *Extract from* Anabolic Steroids are Fool's Gold *by Allan J. Ryan*
> *1981.*

If this is a realistic evaluation then why do so many athletes
persist in taking these drugs? The answer appears to be because
of a mixture of faith and fear. Faith in the evidence that anabolic
steroids[1] do build muscle and increase strength, perhaps a
reasonable idea since 'anabolic' means 'building-up', and fear
that a vital advantage would be lost without them. Having said
this, there would be no reason to ban the use of anabolic
steroids if they had no effect other than to bolster an athlete's
confidence. Something must have prompted their widespread
use in sports and their consequent ban by the IOC Medical
Commission in 1975.

Official testing for anabolic steroids began at the 1976 Montreal Olympics. Perhaps predictably, seven of the eight athletes
disqualified as a result, including two gold medallists, were
weightlifters. Many weightlifters are now resigned to taking
anabolic substances, believing it is impossible to win even a
local championship without them. This pressure pervades all
aspects of sport. American Olympic hammer thrower George

Frenn said: 'I honestly cannot think of one guy, and I know just about all of them personally, who is not using steroids'. The problem is that every competitor is looking for something, anything, that will put him or her among the medal winners. So, when athletes are convinced that a drug works there is enormous pressure to use that drug, irrespective of whether it actually does. Most athletes are absolutely convinced that anabolic steroids are effective in increasing their performance. Despite this, there is a scientific controversy concerning these drugs which can only be understood by reference to the available experimental evidence.

For both men and women, increases in muscle bulk result in greater strength[2]. The theory behind taking anabolic steroids is that they will artificially promote muscle development. The well-defined musculature of the male starts to develop at puberty when the hitherto inactive testes start to produce the 'male hormone' testosterone. This substance courses through the body producing important physiological and psychological changes. The males of other species undergo exactly the same transformation. We know that testosterone is responsible for the changes because castration of immature animals prevents pubertal changes and injections of testosterone can reverse the effects of castration.

The development of bigger muscles is just one of the changes at puberty; this is the *anabolic* action of testosterone. Associated with this are the so-called *androgenic* changes, for example the growth of facial hair and lengthening of the vocal cords which causes the voice to 'break'. In addition to these changes, the ends of growing bones (the epiphyses) start to 'seal', so preventing further lengthening. None of these changes are necessary for reproduction, hence they are referred to as secondary sex characteristics. Those that are important for sexual function, increases in the size of the penis and the initiation of spermatogenesis (sperm production), are called primary sex characteristics.

The powerful anabolic properties of testosterone at puberty have been recognised for over half a century. It is this aspect of the natural hormone that chemists have tried to emulate, and that has attracted the attention of athletes in their search for increased strength. Modern anabolic steroids have effects on muscle growth that are reputedly much greater than that of testosterone (see Table 3.1). Even so, why go to the expense and effort of developing more powerful drugs if testosterone could

TABLE 3.1   Adapted from *Drill's Pharmacology in Medicine* (ed. J. R. DiPalma), McGraw-Hill Inc., 1971

Steroid	Preparation and form	Usual dose	Relative activity	
			Androgenic	Anabolic
Testosterone (Testoral)	10mg sub-lingual tablets	10–30mg/day	1	1
Testosterone propionate (Virormone)	10 + 25mg/ml ampoules	10–50mg twice weekly	1	1
Nandrolone phenpro-pionate (Durabolin)	25mg/ml oil ampoules	25–50mg weekly	1	2.0
Nandrolone decanoate (Deca-Durabolin)	50mg/ml oil ampoules	25–50mg every 3 weeks	1	3.0
Methan-dienone (Dianabol)	5mg tablet	2.5–15mg/day	1	1
Oxymetholone (Anapolon)	5mg tablet	5–15mgday	1	2.0
Stanozolol (Stromba)	5mg tablet	5mg/day	1	3.0

The potency of anabolic steroids is usually compared with that of testosterone. This table shows how certain of the more commonly abused steroids are said to have anabolic activities that exceed their androgenic activities. This should produce fewer of the undesirable 'masculinising' effects (see text for details).

be used instead? There are two reasons for this. First, to be effective testosterone has to be given by injection. If given orally it is transported from the intestine straight to the liver where it is broken down and rendered inactive before it can reach the muscles. It can be given with some success by allowing it to be absorbed from the mouth but this tends to be less satisfactory than an intramuscular injection. Obviously, injections are inconvenient for both doctor and patient, so one reason for developing newer anabolic steroids is that that they can be taken by mouth.

The second reason is that certain of the effects of testosterone are unnecessary and undesirable. Although the practice is now discouraged, anabolic steroids are sometimes used to increase the body weight of children. With powerful androgenic drugs, like testosterone, this can lead to distressing peculiarities such as premature puberty in children, together with masculinising effects in girls. In the latter case girls and women may experience the growth of facial hair, enlargement of the clitoris and deepening of their voices. Some of these effects are irreversible even when the drugs are discontinued. These effects are less of a problem with synthetic anabolic steroids as pharmacologists have designed them to show reduced androgenic activity but increased anabolic activity compared with the prototype testosterone.

All anabolic steroids have some androgenic action and this is often powerful enough to cause considerable problems, for example the stunting of bone growth. Clearly this particular effect is a considerable problem in children. One of the most widely used anabolic steroids, methandienone, was withdrawn in certain countries, in 1982, for this very reason. Anabolic steroids, including testosterone, are used clinically in cases of testicular insufficiency and to promote growth after severely debilitating illnesses. During the Second World War they were given to starvation victims to restore a positive nitrogen balance. In such circumstances anabolic steroids can be very effective but in already healthy individuals, like athletes, their ability to build muscle tissue is disputed.

41

Several different strategies have been used to find out whether anabolic steroids have affected athletic performance. One method is to examine the world's athletics records before and after the advent of these drugs. If steroids are as effective as many people claim we would expect a sharp increase in the rate at which records were broken, compared to the years before their use. This approach has been used by several researchers including Howard Payne, one of Britain's top field event athletes of the 1960s, and a champion of the anti-doping cause. Looking at a variety of events, Payne plotted the average of the world's ten best results for each of the years spanning the introduction of anabolic steroids. Contrary to expectations there seems to be no sudden increase in records for the discus or shot-put, two 'heavy' events almost certain to be affected by truly anabolic drugs. However, all the events Payne examined showed gradual improvements. This makes interpretation of the results difficult. For example, it is impossible to tease-out the advances due to better training methods, from those perhaps caused by steroid use.

A completely different conclusion was reached by Dr. S. Solberg from Tromsø University in Norway. He published data showing the weightlifting results of the ten best lifters at the Norwegian championships over a 20-year period. Between 1962 and 1982 the average body weight of the 'top ten' lifters increased by 18 kg, Solberg claimed this was due to the use of anabolic steroids. Also, in the early 1960s, a time when the sale of anabolic steroids in Norway was low, new records were set at quite a slow pace. However, when sales rocketed between 1968 and 1977 there was a remarkable rise in the rate at which lifting records were broken.

These results might have been due to improved training methods but Solberg prefers to implicate anabolic steroids. Certainly the drugs were used by many Scandinavian athletes in the early 1970s. Surveys showed that in a sample of top male Swedish athletes 31 per cent admitted to taking them. In Norway, the 40 best weightlifters of 1974 were questioned about drug use and 87 per cent of those that volunteered information said they took anabolic steroids. Interestingly, the sale of steroids in Norway has reduced considerably since the mid–seventies. In 1982 sales were less than half those of 1975, perhaps because of the introduction of international anti–doping regulations and testing in 1976. Solberg says that, as a result, the rate of improvement in weightlifting has also dropped, though this claim is hard to substantiate because an important type of lift known as the press was excluded from competition in 1973[3].

Solberg's idea that anabolic steroids augment athletic performance is one which would probably be supported by Sir Roger Bannister, the first man to run a 4-minute mile. In 1973, speaking as chairman of the British Sports Council, Dr. Bannister said: 'Successful testing and elimination of anabolic steroids may, of course, mean that many records set up during the steroid era might not be surpassed for years to come'. Some would point to the Rome European championships as evidence of this. After the shot put event, although the competitors were ranked as predicted, their average performances were down by almost a metre compared with records set prior to the advent of steroid testing.

Payne and Solberg clearly draw different conclusions from previous athletic records. This dichotomy is also apparent from the controlled studies that have investigated the effects of anabolic steroids on strength and body weight. The results of these studies show that anabolic steroids do not always produce clear increases in weight or performance. The reason for this might lie in Allan Ryan's statement which opens this chapter. He is very careful to point out that 'steroids will not contribute significantly to gains in *lean muscle* bulk or muscle strength in *healthy* young adult males'. (emphasis added). Anabolic steroids were intended for use in malnourished convalescing patients, and few sportsmen or women fall into this category. In other words, according to Dr. Ryan, anabolic steroids may have minimal effects on healthy athletes.

In his article 'Anabolic steroids are fool's gold', Allan Ryan reviewed 25 studies carried out between 1965 and 1977[4]. Most

43

of these measured strength changes by noting the weight achieved in standard 'power' lifts but also looked at changes in body weight and muscle circumference. Ryan found that 13 of these studies showed no effect of anabolic steroids on ability to lift weights but the remaining ones did. The latter were dismissed by Dr. Ryan on the basis of their poor design, though we feel that many of his criticisms are unjustified. There certainly have been *some* well-designed experiments which showed clear improvements in strength after treatment with anabolic steroids. For example, Dr. David Freed, from Manchester University, and his colleagues used 13 experienced weightlifters in a double-blind trial of methandienone[5]. In a double-blind trial neither the clinician nor the athlete know whether they are receiving steroid or 'dummy' tablets (placebo). The substances are simply coded and their identity kept secret until the experiment is over, and this prevents the doctor or subject from influencing the results. Sometimes, in these trials, it is obvious to the athlete that he is taking steroids because of the effects on body weight or performance. In such cases the subjects have been known to abscond from the trial taking their free samples with them.

Dr. Freed used six standard strength exercises and found that, over a 6-week period of treatment, methandienone increased lifting capacity by between 0.3 and 13 per cent. However, the results were very variable. Some lifters showed no greater improvement than those taking placebo where performance improved by between 0.3 and 2.3 per cent. Body weight also increased in the steroid treated athletes. Interestingly, the dose, 10mg or 25 mg per day, was unimportant in deciding the degree of improvement: the higher dose was no more effective than the lower. After the 6-week treatment period, body weight returned to its normal level but, Dr. Freed claimed, the increase in strength *remained*. The implication of this is immense. An athlete might be able to take steroids during training then withdraw early enough to produce a negative urine test at the time of competition, yet still benefit from an unfair doping advantage. Similar results were found by a group of Finnish scientists. Drs. Alen, Hakkinen and Komi studied a number of top-class power athletes who were self-administering high doses of anabolic steroids[6]. In addition to showing increased performance on certain strength tests, these men continued to improve their performance during the subsequent 6-week withdrawal period.

Clearly, the results of David Freed's work show that there is a lot of individual variation in the response to anabolic steroids. This is probably an important factor in determining the outcome of such studies and may account for some of the confusion over the effects of these drugs. It seems that only a proportion of people show clear improvements in performance as a result of steroid treatment.

Other factors could help explain the negative opinions of scientists such as Allan Ryan. For example, because they are human experiments, the studies conducted on athletes have to be approved by local ethical commitees. In order to get approval the clinician conducting the study has to agree to use doses that are proven to be safe. Consequently, most of the reported trials have used doses that are well below those normally used by the athletes as part of their training programme. Hence it might be that much higher doses of steroids have the anabolic effect that athletes claim, whereas scientists are unable to show this with their lower doses. In his autobiography, Britain's most successful shot-putter Geoff Capes[7] described how athletes responded when one of his rivals, Jeff Teale, revealed that he had taken anabolic steroids at a dose of half a tablet a day; a reasonable dose by medical standards:

The world's throwers fell about laughing. It was like saying he had drunk two bottles of milk for all the effect it could have had on him. But that was what it was like in the late 1960s and early 1970s. Everybody was experimenting. It was all trial and error.

Over a 5-year period Teale did actually increase his consumption of steroids (see Chapter 1) but Capes' comment illustrates how athletes ridicule the use of therapeutic doses.

In addition to dose differences, the procedures for steroid use by athletes vary markedly to those used in clinical studies. Many weightlifters, for example, use a process called 'stacking', where different types of steroid are used concurrently. The athlete may start a drugs programme by using a low dose of an oral anabolic steroid. The dose would be increased after a week or so and supplemented with a weekly injection of one of the long-acting steroids such as nandrolone decanoate. Over the next few weeks the doses and frequency of these treatments would be increased. A month before competition the athlete might be taking about ten times the therapeutic dose of oral steroids, plus perhaps six or eight times the therapeutic dose of injectable long-acting steroids. In an attempt to avoid detection, for the few weeks prior to competition the synthetic drugs would be dropped, to be replaced by testosterone[8].

The vast majority of weightlifters who believe in the effectiveness of anabolic steroids, the 'bulk bomb', think that hard training and correct diet are also needed to achieve results. Clinical studies verify this to some extent. In his excellent article 'Anabolic steroids and athletics' James Wright discusses the actions of steroids on experienced and inexperienced subjects[9]. After reviewing studies on the latter (i.e. those who did not train with weights *before* the study) he concluded that:

> inexperienced weight trainers, using therapeutic doses of anabolic hormones could expect a weight gain amounting to approximately 1.5kg, over what could be expected from training alone. The comparison of the weight gain remains open to question, particularly since, under these circumstances, strength will probably not be affected to the extent that body weight is affected.

Even with short-term weight training and protein supplements anabolic steroids had little effect on strength or lean muscle mass in these subjects. In weightlifters who trained on a regular basis (i.e. three or four times weekly), to near maximum capacity, the results are rather different. The outcome of these studies led Wright to conclude:

> The data on strength indicate that anabolic steroids may indeed be ergogenic when taken by experienced weight trainers in conjunction with a program of heavy-resistance exercise. The reason for the different findings compared to inexperienced subjects is unknown.

However, the results were far from consistent, and in the end Wright was forced to agree with Allan Ryan that overall there was 'about an even split on the effects of steroids on strength enhancement'. Another eminent sports-scientist, Professor David Lamb of Purdue University, Indiana, and former president of the American College of Sports Medicine, drew similar conclusions[10].

Overall, the conclusions from studies such as these have led to the opinion stated in most sports medicine textbooks: anabolic steroids have not been shown to improve performance. Since most athletes do not share this opinion it is our experience that scientists run the risk of losing credibility with the layman unless they can suggest reasons for the discrepancy. We have already pointed to dose differences as one possibility, but a 1984 review by Drs. Haupt and Rovere identifies certain design differences between studies which also shed some light on the disagreement[11]. They agreed with Wright that experienced athletes training to near maximum capacity *before* the trial were an essential requirement for the study. They also found that the way strength changes were measured was also important, as was the maintenence of a high-protein diet. Generally Drs. Haupt and Rovere found that, under these circumstances, anabolic steroids consistently produced an increase in strength – an observation which might help to restore the athlete's faith in science!

In addition to a direct effect on muscle strength, under certain circumstances, there are other reasons why athletes might risk taking these potentially harmful drugs. First, athletes have an over-inflated idea of the potency of steroids. Second, bodybuilders are 'image conscious' and take steroids for cosmetic reasons. Third, and perhaps most important, they are taken to allow longer, harder training periods which in themselves could improve performance.

However, if athletes are wrong about the potency of anabolic steroids then scientists must take some of the blame. Anabolic steroids were developed after work was published by Drs. Kochakian and Murlin in 1935[12]. The conclusion of this was that testosterone increased body weight in castrated male dogs. Further research was conducted to develop 'testosterone like' substances without the undesirable, masculinising (androgenic) effects. In order to discover potentially useful substances a simple assay method had to be developed to determine their potency. One might think that any skeletal muscle could be used for this, one could simply measure the weight gained by the muscle as a result of drug treatment. It may come as a surprise to learn that scientists had great difficulty finding such muscles. The only one considered suitable was the rat's levator ani, a small muscle which forms part of the male reproductive system.

In retrospect, it seems ridiculous that no-one questioned the reason why skeletal muscles (those that move limbs) were not responsive to testosterone as Kochakian and Murlin had suggested. A large number of anabolic steroids were developed and their potency was compared with testosterone using the rat levator ani test. This produced information like that presented in Table 3.1. Many athletes decide which steroid to take on the basis of these potencies, so stanozolol (Stromba) and nandrolone (Durabolin) are favourite choices. In fact, there is no evidence that any of these orally active, synthetic drugs is more potent than injections of testosterone propionate in increasing muscle mass.

The results of experiments on animals do not always parallel those on humans. It is worth stressing that many scientists are convinced that so-called anabolic steroids have no real anabolic effects in animals. If this is so, it may also help to explain the inconsistent results found in athletes. It is also worth pointing out that commercial meat animals usually do not gain weight when treated with male hormones. Surprisingly, female (oestrogenic) substances are normally used for this purpose[13].

Many strength athletes claim to develop bigger muscles while undergoing heavy training supplemented with steroids. Often their muscles grow so fast that their skin growth cannot keep pace and they show 'stretch marks'. A lot of experiments support the idea that anabolic steroids increase muscle circumference; what they cannot agree on is whether this represents an increase in *normal* muscle tissue. There are some scientists who say steroids are able to enhance the build-up of normal muscle proteins; however, many would agree with Professor G. R. Hervey, a Leeds University physiologist, who thinks that steroids increase muscle circumference by promoting a rapid intake of water and tissue salts. In other words, anabolic steroids cause muscles to become 'bloated'. Experiments that have investigated the nitrogen and mineral composition of steroid-treated muscles support this theory to some extent[14].

Clearly, this muscle 'inflation' enhances the appearance of bodybuilders but it may be of little use in strength events. Having said this, there may be a powerful psychological effect of body image on performance. If an athlete knows he is getting bigger, for whatever reason, this factor alone could improve his athletic ability. Certainly, the knowledge that he/she is taking steroids is important in deciding final performance. Several studies have shown that when athletes are given dummy injections or tablets, but *told* they are getting anabolic steroids, they may out-perform those correctly told they are receiving placebo and can often equal the performance of those given steroids.

The final point concerns muscular endurance. Heavy exercise causes the production of cortisol, itself a steroid, from the adrenal cortex (the outer part of the adrenal gland). As one of its actions this hormone causes the catabolism, or breakdown, of muscle proteins. Some physiologists believe that anabolic steroids block the effects of cortisol, reducing muscle breakdown so increasing their size. Anabolic steroids might also prevent the destruction of cortisol by the liver, which would raise the level of cortisol in the blood.

Excessively high blood cortisol produces some interesting effects which might explain some casual observations of typical 'heavy' athletes. First, the shape of athletes has changed over the last 20 or 30 years. Weightlifters and throwers of the pre-steroid era had lean, well-defined physiques. Modern athletes have more of a fattened, 'puffy' appearance. High cortisol secretion can produce this effect; it occurs naturally in the state known as Cushing's disease (see Chapter 6). Also, many athletes say they use anabolic steroids because they can train harder, more intensively and for longer periods. Excessive cortisol in the blood might make this possible by increasing the availability of glucose and reducing muscle fatigue. This is interesting because, as already suggested, it could be that anabolic steroids might have no direct effects on muscle tissue, but simply allow more exercise which then causes greater muscle growth. These effects might explain why steroids are taken by runners. Reduced recovery times mean that more frequent, intensive training is possible, enabling athletes to compete more often. Following her withdrawal from the 1980 Moscow Olympics, in protest at the reinstatement of three athletes given 'life' bans for steroid abuse, British runner Christine Benning commented:

> Those girls were running the equivalent of the British record three times a week, and at the time I couldn't understand how they could do it because I knew if I did, I'd get injured. When it came out they'd been taking steroids, of course, everything became clear.

It seems ludicrous that 'clean' athletes should have to forsake their own chance of victory in order to make a point.

Some scientists believe that psychological effects of sex hormones could be responsible for the improvements in performance claimed by steroid users. Popular opinion is that testosterone-like substances increase aggression; consequently, anabolic steroids have also been endowed with this property. In lower animals testosterone is needed for the expression of hostility but in highly social animals, especially primates, the effects are much more complex. Social interaction is an important factor in primates because an animal's position in the dominance hierarchy or 'pecking order' partly determines its production of testosterone. So the dominant male often produces more testosterone and is more aggressive *because* it is the dominant male, not vice versa. Nevertheless, androgenic substances certainly have some potential to increase aggression and if anabolic steroids also have this ability then they might be used to evoke the aggressive-rage syndrome that certain competitors consider advantageous. American footballers seem to be particularly prone to this sort of abuse. In addition to using high doses of amphetamines to induce paranoid rage (see Chapter 2), they are also heavy users of anabolic steroids. A report in *Sports Illustrated* (May 1985) suggested that 95 per cent of professional American footballers have tried anabolic steroids at some time and 75 per cent are regular users. One player admitted to spending over £2000 a year on drugs just to stay in the game. Clearly some footballers would use anabolic steroids to increase their bulk but, in view of their suggested effects on aggression, they could also be used for psychological reasons.

Athletes, especially those in the 'heavy' events, consume enormous amounts of food. For example, it has been reported that the daily food intake of athletes in the 1936 Olympic games was over 7000 kilocalories (kcal). This was about 3 times the average intake of the time! This tradition has persisted. American athletes in 1976 still ate almost twice the national average. There is a commonly held belief that these quantities are needed, especially when taking anabolic steroids, to maintain or increase muscle tissue. Since protein constitutes muscle, athletes tend to include a disproportionate amount of protein in their diets, usually in the form of eggs, meat and commercial 'supplements'. As protein-rich diets are an expensive way of eating it would be useful to know whether they helped. Evidence from

51

research on athletes not taking steroids shows that high caloric intake and high protein intake are unnecessary. For example, even long-distance runners who run over 170km a week probably need no more than 4000kcal daily. Since the average daily intake for non-athletes is 2100kcal for women and 2700kcal for men, this need can be met by a relatively modest increase in dietary intake.

As far as protein is concerned, it has been estimated that our daily requirement is about 0.6 g for every kilogram of body weight. In heavy exercise this need is increased to between 1 and 2 g/kg. Analysis of a typical American diet shows that even sedentary people take in more than this. Athletes eat two or three times the normal quantity, so their protein intake greatly exceeds their requirements. Anabolic steroids are supposed to have their muscle-building effects by causing the retention of nitrogen from dietary protein; that is they shift the body's 'nitrogen balance'. Although no hard evidence exists to show that a high-protein diet assists this process, it might when combined with the massive doses of steroids which are used by many athletes.

One of the ways by which sporting authorities deter athletes from using anabolic steroids is through placing great emphasis on side effects. In practice this may have little effect; the possibility of immediate gains in performance often outweigh the risk of undesirable effects. These side effects are often very long-term and may even go completely unnoticed by the majority of athletes. As Ron Pickering, BBC commentator and coach, has said: 'It's no use trying to scare them by saying their balls will drop off'.

The father of synthetic anabolic steroids Dr. John B. Ziegler, himself a strength athlete, knew the dangers of steroid use. After collaborating with the pharmaceutical company Ciba-Geigy on the production of methandienone (Dianabol) in the 1950s he became disenchanted with the way a useful therapeutic drug was abused by his fellow sportsmen. Ziegler came to condemn the use of anabolic steroids in athletics partly because they represented an unhealthy aspect of sport, but also because of their side effects. Weightlifters and bodybuilders, the biggest (no pun intended) offenders in the steroid stakes, are often vaguely aware of the sorts of problems they might expect but few athletes admit to experiencing them. One person who helped to increase awareness of the side effects was the Swedish discus-thrower Ricky Bruch. Bruch was a bronze medallist at the 1972 Olympic Games and in September 1978 he admitted on British television that he had started taking steroids 10 years earlier. Since then he had suffered a fractured vertebra, had six knee operations, internal problems and a mental breakdown. He claimed that these were the result of massive doses of anabolic steroids and he urged young athletes not to follow his example. Bruch's case is probably a little extreme but the side effects should not be underestimated.

To describe the side effects of anabolic steroids we first need to explain what how these substances affect the body. Figure 3.1 shows their major sites of action.

Before going into descriptions of specific health risks it is important to point out a general problem associated with the abuse of any illicit drugs. Because they are used without medical supervision, illicit injectable substances are often of suspect origin and are administered in less than ideal circumstances. Disposable syringes are supposed to be discarded after use but, because drug users have limited access to them, they are often used more than once and by different people. This practice has contributed enormously to the spread of certain diseases in those people who inject, for example, heroin. Equally at risk are those athletes who share syringes for the administration of long-acting anabolic steroids. Although acquired immune deficiency syndrome (AIDS) is widely considered a problem associated with homosexuality, it is also common among drug addicts who share syringes. Athletes who dose themselves with injectable steroids also run this risk. One case of AIDS in a weightlifter has already been reported in a man who had no history of homosexuality or hard drug-abuse[15]. He admitted to sharing syringes with his fellow bodybuilders but stopped this when, 2 years earlier, he had contracted hepatitis B.

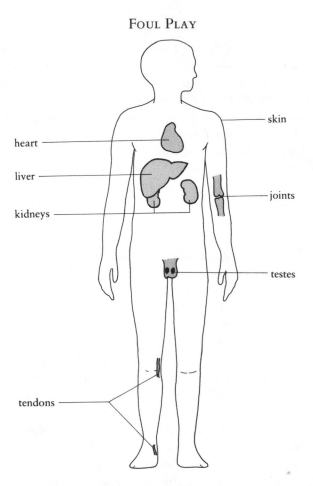

heart

liver

kidneys

skin

joints

testes

tendons

FIGURE 3.1 Schematic diagram of the body showing the points where anabolic steroids are known to act and, potentially, cause damage. See text for details.

Anabolic steroids can, in large doses and with prolonged use, produce a 'puffy' appearance of the face and trunk. Another, more common, problem is acne, which many athletes consider to be a tell-tale sign of steroid abuse. This occurs, as it does in adolescent males, because androgens stimulate the activity of the sebaceous glands in the skin which leads to the oiliness responsible for acne. In addition, athletes may develop large

54

inflamed follicles, especially on the upper back. These eventually burst and become reinfected if steroid use continues.

Steroid sex hormones have been implicated in cardiovascular disease. Hypertension (high blood pressure) and coronary heart disease are the biggest killers in the West so their importance should not be underestimated. Sex steroids may place an unnecessary load on the heart through two main actions:

First, they increase atherosclerosis (furring-up of the arteries with fatty deposits) perhaps by reducing the blood levels of certain lipids that help to remove these deposits. One study estimated that if the levels of these protective lipids (so-called high density lipids), dropped by 10 per cent this would increase the chances of a heart attack by 25 per cent. Some athletes have been found to have high density lipid concentrations so low that their chances of a heart attack may be doubled.

Second, steroids also cause considerable salt retention. This causes an excessive amount of water to be retained in order to compensate. In turn, the increased fluid retention forces up the blood pressure. As any plumber knows, the power required to pump water through a central heating system is determined by the diameter of the pipes and the backpressure of the system. The cardiovascular system is very similar and failure of the pump, in this case the heart, can occur prematurely due to atherosclerosis or hypertension.

Oral contraceptives also increase the risk of cardiovascular disease but, statistically, the risks are minimal compared with the dangers associated with pregnancy, the possible consequence of not taking them. In athletics, anabolic steroids are not taken to avoid becoming pregnant, or to avoid any other potentially dangerous condition. They are also consumed in much higher doses than oral contraceptives, so the risks are both unnecessary and considerably greater.

As with any drug, steroids have most side effects on the physiological systems involved in their metabolism, excretion and transport. The liver has an essential role in the metabolism of many chemicals and its function is considerably affected by steroids. The commonest steroid-induced liver problem is cho-

55

lestatic jaundice, a progressive reduction in liver functioning which, although potentially fatal, usually disappears within 3 months of steroid withdrawal. One of the symptoms of this is a yellow tinge to the skin caused by the presence of bile pigments in the blood when they should have been rendered excretable by the liver. Less frequent, but more serious, are the possibilities of liver cancer (hepatoma) and peliosis (where blood-filled spaces appear in the liver). Both these are more common in athletes who had a history of liver disease before taking steroids, but there is an alarming increase in their incidence in athletes previously known to be healthy.

The first case of an athlete dying from hepatoma after steroid abuse was reported by Dr. Wylie Overly from Pennsylvania. An anonymous 26-year-old weightlifter took anabolic steroids intermittently for 4 years despite knowing about the possible cancer link. He weighed 180 lb (81.6 kg) when cancer was diagnosed but only 100 lb (45.3 kg) when he died 4 months later. There is no proof that anabolic steroids caused the disease but as Dr. Overly said 'it's pretty well established that these drugs are carcinogenic, and it certainly has to be suspected'.

Anabolic steroids are based on the chemical structure of testosterone (see Figure 3.2). However, there are certain impor-

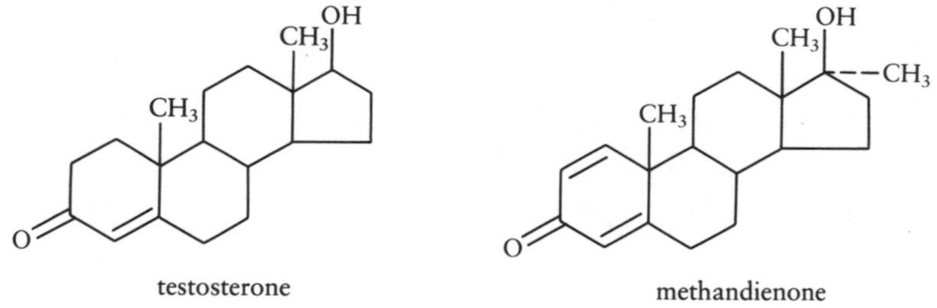

testosterone

methandienone

FIGURE 3.2 The chemical structures of all anabolic steroids are similar to that of testosterone. In order that they become active after oral dosing, the basic structure must be modified to include an additional chemical group at the C_{17} position.

tant differences which affect the incidence of certain side effects. In order for anabolic steroids to be active by the oral route pharmacologists have had to modify the basic structure of testosterone (which is only active by injection). Methandienone (Dianabol), for example, has an additional chemical grouping on the C_{17} position of the molecule. If this group were not present then the drug would be rapidly metabolised and rendered inactive by the liver. Without this C_{17} substitution the steroid would not be orally active; the price for this convenience is that all orally active anabolic steroids are more likely to cause liver damage.

Oral contraceptive steroids share these side-effects since they too are C_{17} substituted, but hepatic damage is rare unless the steroids are taken in very high doses. Even at clinical doses oral contraceptives are taken at only one tenth of the dose of anabolic agents. As with the cardiovascular effects, the real danger of liver damage is to athletes who take amounts greatly in excess of the normal dose.

The liver and kidneys are often damaged by abuse of any drug simply because these organs are responsible for its metabolism and excretion. It is not possible to identify a causal relationship between steroid use and kidney damage because there is insufficient evidence available at present.

In his recent book *Death in the Locker Room*, Bob Goldman writes a moving account of the premature demise of one of America's leading strength athletes[16]. This man, together with the 1958 AAU Mr. America Tom Sansone, died from Wilm's tumour, a cancer of the kidney. Although two cases may not appear particularly significant, certain aspects of these strongly implicate anabolic steroids. First, both men were known to have taken anabolic steroids during their bodybuilding careers. Second, Wilm's tumour usually appears in the embryo and is detected before the age of 8 in 90 per cent of cases; apparently only *150* examples have ever been recorded in adults. The chances of two of those 150 having a history of weightlifting and anabolic steroids abuse must be very slim indeed, unless the drugs were in some way related to the disorder.

Anabolic steroids were once used to promote growth in underdeveloped children; their use in such cases is now discouraged. Medical opinion has changed because of evidence that anabolic steroids cause premature sealing of the ends of growing bones. The result is that bone growth stops. Clearly this, despite any overall anabolic effect, would hinder the child's development rather than assist it. Children are not the only population at risk. The long bones of the legs, for example, do not stop growing until about the age of 20; others of the chest and backbone grow for some years after this. Anabolic steroid use in adolescent athletes seems to be an increasing problem, especially in the United States; how many of these Olympic hopefuls realise they are actually reducing their chances of successful future competition?

In those individuals who experience increases in their performance as a result of taking anabolic steroids there is a danger of tendon damage. Tendons are tough pieces of tissue that anchor muscles to the bones they move. Damage is particularly pronounced in weightlifters who dramatically increase their lifting poundage. The abnormally high strain that is put upon the tendons in weightlifting is exacerbated by the performance increase which might result from steroid abuse. In such cases the tendons have no time to adapt to the rapid increase in power of the muscles and consequently can be severely damaged.

A great deal has been said about anabolic steroids and the male reproductive system; much of it is unfounded but some of it is undoubtedly true and should be seriously considered. Anabolic steroids reduce normal testosterone production, often to the levels seen in castrated males; in addition spermatogenesis (sperm production) frequently ceases. What is less certain is the risk of long-term damage to testicular function that may occur due to continuous steroid treatment. Testosterone is produced by the testes; normally, this is limited to between 5 and 10mg per day. A chemical from the hypothalamus at the base of the brain (luteinising hormone releasing hormone) stimulates the pituitary gland to produce gonadotrophins, luteinising hormone (LH) and follicle stimulating hormone (FSH). LH is

58

carried in the bloodstream to the testes where it stimulates testosterone secretion. FSH is also active in the testes where it is responsible, jointly with testosterone, for spermatogenesis. When blood levels of testosterone become too high this is detected by the pituitary and hypothalamus which switch off the production of gonadotrophins, just as a thermostat switches off the heating when the temperature reaches a critical level (see Figure 3.3).

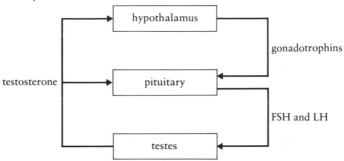

FIGURE 3.3 Schematic diagram showing the control of testicular function by the hypothalamus and pituitary. The hypothalamus produces gonadotrophins which stimulate the pituitary, this releases follicle stimulating hormone (FSH) and luteinising hormone (LH) which cause testosterone release from the testes. High levels of testosterone inhibit the release of FSH and LH.

However, the detection mechanisms that monitor the levels of testosterone cannot tell the difference between natural testosterone and testosterone-like substances that are injected or swallowed. Consequently, when anabolic steroids are taken they disrupt the control mechanisms. This reduces natural testosterone output and, as a result, inhibits sperm production. The problem is that without testosterone to maintain its functioning there is a danger that the male reproductive system may waste away. On the basis of this argument many authorities, including Professors Raymond Brooks of St. Thomas's Hospital, London and Arnold Beckett of the IOC Medical Commission, believe we are producing a field of 'chemically castrated' athletes.

As far as we are aware, no athlete has been found to exhibit *permanent* changes to the reproductive system as a result of anabolic steroid use. Although normal hormone levels may be low during steroid use they return to normal after the drug is discontinued. However, few studies have been conducted on athletes who have taken steroids for long periods. Most have looked at administration for only a few months, whereas many weightlifters take them for years. For the present, the question of irreversible changes must remain open. but it is conceivable that anabolic steroids could cause permanent damage.

That anabolic steroids suppress normal testicular function is undeniable, but what effect does this have on sexual perfor-mance? While there is a clear relationship between the increase in testosterone levels and the onset of sexual development at puberty, control of human sexual behaviour is exquisitely com-plex and not dependent on any single hormone. Research in animals shows that artificial reductions in testosterone levels produced by castration will quickly cause sterility; some time later sexual activity will cease. For example, male rats will continue to copulate for up to 5 months after castration even though their blood testosterone levels drop to zero within hours. When sexual activity stops, injections of testosterone will usually restore fertility and potency. This parallels the human case where men have been castrated either for sexual offences, through accidents or because of surgery. In these men, impotence may take years to develop but again is restored by several weeks of testosterone therapy. The time course and outcome of these events appears to depend on the amount of precastration sexual experience more than anything else.

The discrepancy between absolute testosterone blood levels and sexual activity probably arises because of the way testoster-one works. It has at least two actions on sexual behaviour. First, it maintains the physical structure of the sex organs through the action of one of its breakdown products; without this substance the sensitivity of the penis is reduced and this can markedly affect sexual activity. Such structural changes may take months to appear after castration. Second, testosterone acts in several

60

parts of the central nervous system to increase libido, the sexual urge. In the latter respect androgens such as testosterone also seem to perform the same function in women (see Chapter 4).

In humans the complexity of the sexual response precludes any simple explanation of the importance of testosterone. It is probably most accurate to say that male sexual behaviour is related to testosterone in an all-or-none, rather than a graded, fashion. If enough testosterone is present then sexual activity will proceed as normal; if production drops below a critical level then it will stop. Clinical investigations of testosterone output in men who self-administer steroids show that most subjects have abnormally low blood testosterone levels (i.e. below the accepted range of 400–1000 ng/ml). It is not possible to tell if the lower limit of this range is 'critical' in relation to sexual activity; for some men it may be. Whether athletes experience reductions in libido or potency is difficult to ascertain. Anecdotal reports usually claim that no such side effects are found. However, the validity of these are questionable since few men would admit to having a low sex drive. More rigorous interrogation often reveals that while some men feel a reduction in their libido others show more interest in sex.

THE DETECTION OF ANABOLIC STEROIDS

Until 1973 no suitable detection method was available for the large-scale screening of urine samples for anabolic steroids, the main reason being that the drug dose taken is very small and when this is distributed throughout the body it is present in only minute quantities. At that time the analytical techniques were not sufficiently sensitive to detect them. However, in 1973, Professor Raymond Brooks of St. Thomas' Hospital London announced a breakthrough in the detection of anabolic steroids; his team had been working on a new method for the previous 3 years with sponsorship from the British Sports Council. As a result of this advance, in April 1975 the IOC Medical Commission decided to include anabolic steroids on the list of banned drugs. The method was tested at the New Zealand Commonwealth Games of 1974, but no penalties were imposed on the nine offenders (out of 55 tested) because steroids had not yet been officially banned. It was in 1976 at the Montreal Olympics that serious testing was first carried out.

The method developed by Brooks is a two-stage process combining the techniques of radioimmunoassay and gas chromatography/mass spectrometry (see Appendix C for details). The whole method is very sensitive; it has been claimed that positive urine tests have been found several months after the last dose of anabolic steroids. This may be true for long-acting injectable drugs such as nandrolone decanoate (Decadurabolin), but the shorter-acting steroids are much more difficult to detect; with oral anabolic steroids, for example, detection may be impossible only a few days after the last dose. In any case many athletes claim to know when to stop taking steroids in order to produce a negative test result. The information that was available to British shot-putter Geoff Capes[7] is probably typical of athletes who are faced with the problem of tests at competition:

> When Ilona Slupianek, the East German who won the 1978 European gold medal and the 1980 Olympic title, was convicted, we were told it was because her doctor did not use a long enough needle. He had injected the drug into the body fat instead of the muscle and it had been retained in her body for longer than it should have been. So the usual clearance period of two to four weeks was not enough, and she was caught. And that is the only way the testers catch anybody – when the athletes make a mistake.

Athletes are enterprising people; as soon as detection methods are developed for one anabolic agent they move onto another. Professor Arnold Beckett of the IOC Medical Commission admitted: 'After we discovered a test for the anabolic steroids the athletes regrouped and considered what to do. They found testosterone. It's a war, and we are facing a whole new battle.' Testosterone, which of course is produced normally by the body, is being used increasingly by athletes to prolong the effects of earlier courses of synthetic steroids. This way they can leave ample time for their bodies to 'flush-out' all traces of synthetic steroids yet maintain the anabolic effect by 'topping-up' with testosterone. With synthetic anabolic steroids the IOC ruling is clear: the detection of any amount, however small, constitutes a positive result. The problem with testosterone is the fact that it occurs naturally in the body, so the detection methods have to distinguish between naturally produced and administered testosterone. This is not easy. Interpretation of the results of this type of test leaves much room for doubt and, since there is so much at stake, officials must be very cautious about declaring a positive result[17]. The same problem applies to tests for caffeine – how much is too much? Tests for high levels of both testosterone and caffeine were introduced by the IOC in time for the 1984 Los Angeles Olympics.

Current research by Irving Dardik, United States Olympic Commitee Sports Medicine Chairman, is aimed at increasing the body's production of testosterone by natural means. Levels of testosterone are not constant and Dardik claims that by training when testosterone production is highest, the athlete can achieve increases in performance greater than those produced by anabolic steroids, without the side effects. Dardik says that exercising when testosterone levels are high causes even more testosterone release. He claims that this technique will 'without question' eradicate the use of anabolic steroids. The problem for the vast majority of athletes is that they have no facilities for measuring their own testosterone output. So, despite Dardik's enthusiasm, it is likely that the convenience of a syringe or bottle of tablets will continue to prove a more attractive alternative.

Dr. Dardik may have succeeded in boosting testosterone production through exercise but increasing numbers of athletes are doing this artificially by using human chorionic gonadotrophin (HCG). This substance is produced by the developing placenta through which a baby derives its nourishment, and is

63

obtained from pregnant women's urine. HCG has a therapeutic use in certain types of female infertility. In men its action is basically that of LH in that it causes testosterone production from the testes (see Figure 3.3). Professor Arnold Beckett realised the impact that HCG and growth hormone would have on international sport. Prior to the 1984 Olympic Games he spoke of the 'huge gap' these drugs had opened-up in dope control: 'If we don't do something that gap will remain. It is not too late. We should ban both drugs'. For those games his words were to no avail; the authorities are notoriously slow to respond to the challenge of new doping practices.

Despite the scientific controversy all the weightlifters we know are firm believers in the effectiveness of anabolic steroids. In the battle for credibility the scientist often loses to those professing 'grass roots' experience. So ultimately an athlete will listen to his fellow sportsmen, partly because he wants to believe that steroids work, but also because a personal account of their efficacy is far more convincing than the results of a detached scientific study. Discussions with weightlifters who have used steroids often reveal a long series of tales describing men who, after years of training, were unable to improve. After a couple of weeks on the 'bomb' they were lifting much greater poundages. Faced with this sort of evidence what chance does the sport stand? Wally Holland, secretary of the British Amateur Weightlifting Association (BAWLA), is aware of the lure of steroids: 'Let's face it people are all looking for short cuts to being champions – and that's what taking steroids is all about: cheating, just downright cheating'.

The official line contrasts sharply with the ugly scenes that have recently taken place out of the public eye. In 1983 a disillusioned weightlifter, Ken Smith, was suspended indefinitely by BAWLA. He claimed that BAWLA did not encourage an active detection policy and said he had testimonials describing how officials have offered to 'accidentally' lose urine samples from top competitors. Smith's intention was to set up his own Natural Weightlifting Assocation in opposition to BAWLA; as a result the suspension was imposed 'for malicious conduct designed to bring the sport into disrepute'. When he threatened BAWLA with high court action he was reinstated, only to be resuspended when he continued to speak out. Mr. Smith remained defiant: 'The suspension is a way of shutting me up. It won't work.'

Only a year later the same thing happened to BAWLA's official registrar of records, Tony Cook. He had used his weightlifting newsletter *Backhang Gazette* to anger BAWLA officials and was ordered to attend a disciplinary hearing. When he failed to appear he was suspended with no right of appeal. Cook was simply telling the truth when he said:

> Today, 16-year-olds are making lifts that 15 years ago grown men were unable to achieve. Don't tell me that school milk has made all that difference. The fact is that drugs are now taken at every level in the sport, and every club in Britain has a tale to tell.

As former registrar of records, Cook should know what he is talking about.

Wally Holland expresses understandable despair at the way athletes beat the system; like others he is well aware of the continual exploitation of loopholes in detection methods. While it is true that weightlifters are a driving force behind new techniques in drug abuse, anabolic steroids remain the most commonly abused drugs in sport. The final word rests with Dr. David Cowan, assistant director of the Drug Control and Testing Centre at Chelsea:

> The mechanism *does* exist for controlling drugs. The laboratory tests are effective. What is required is a commitment from these sports to more frequent testing in and out of competition.

4

DRUGS AND THE FEMALE ATHLETE

That is not a normal physiological female body. I've treated Olympic female athletes in 34 countries but I've never seen a body like that. I can truthfully say that I think there is something chemically different about her physical make-up and it hasn't come from weight-lifting.

Dr. Leroy Perry, Los Angeles chiropracter,
talking about Czech middle-distance runner Jarmila Kratochvilova.

This statement embodies the thoughts of many people when they first see muscular women athletes like Kratochvilova. However, there is a growing school of enlightened opinion which views this as Victorian resistance to the relentless upsurge of women in sport. Successful female athletes often have physiques that put many men to shame. The fact that they do makes most of us defensive, yet there is no reason why women should not have a powerful physique. We should ask whether our social constraints regarding the female 'ideal' be allowed to dictate the development of women's sport. Instead of questioning the physical and chemical make-up of Jarmila Kratochvilova perhaps Dr. Perry should have scrutinised his own male chauvinism. Having said this, there is something about the bodies of women such as runner Kratochvilova and weightlifter Bev Francis which tests the mettle of even the most liberal-minded people.

In most respects it is acknowledged that women have the

potential to be as good as men; the fact that they often do not realise their abilities can be a product of the way society treats them. Even the law is not impartial when it comes to women and sport; section 44 of the 1975 British Sex Discrimination Act says that discrimination is not unlawful in sports where the average woman is disadvantaged physically compared to the average man. The fact that women should be allowed the freedom to choose their sports does not seem to be important[1]. This is not an international problem since many countries (e.g. USA) do not have such severe restrictions; however the Olympic Committee has ruled that certain events should not be open to women. Today, the hammer throw, triple jump, steeplechase and pole vault are all men-only events; until 1984 so were track events longer than 1500m. This may still seem unfair but the number of women's events is gradually increasing.

In ancient times the Olympics were men-only events, women were not even allowed to watch; this rule was enforced with capital punishment. A similar attitude was adopted by Baron Pierre de Coubertin, father of the 'modern' Olympics, who said that women would only participate over his dead body. After he stood down as President more enlightened opinions prevailed and women were allowed to compete in some of the events at the 1928 Olympics at Amsterdam. However, even this was not plain sailing since after the 800m race several of the competitors collapsed from exhaustion, an incident that antifeminists used very effectively against the pioneers of women's sport. They managed to cajole the male-dominated IAAF and IOC into banning women's events of over 200m, on the grounds that participants were sure to damage their health. Consequently the women's 400 and 800m races were not reintroduced until 1964 and 1960 respectively.

Despite the antiquated ideals of the IOC, women are rapidly pushing through physical and psychological barriers to become a real force in modern sport. Women's athletics records are being set at a much faster rate than those of men. If trends continue then women's marathon times will equal those of men by the end of the century. Women currently swim at speeds comparable to those of men in 1970 and their middle-distance running times are now on a par with those of men of the 1930s. According to Dr. Paul Wade[2], consultant to the US Olympic Committee Elite Program, the women's high jump world record has improved by 40 per cent over the last 60 years compared with only 29 per cent by men in over 100 years. As Dr. Wade points out, this discrepancy cannot continue. Women's sport is still in its infancy and only undergoing phenomenal advances in performance because women are learning to train in a way that was previously denied them; perhaps quite soon their rates of improvement will fall to those of men. Ultimately, sheer physical strength will mark the difference between male and female athletic capability, although several endurance events may favour the woman's more efficient fat-burning processes and her ability to control body temperature without excessive water loss through sweating. Given appropriate encouragement and facilities women should eventually compete on equal terms with men in those events where greater total strength is not important.

Inevitably, our male-dominated Western societies will be forced to welcome a faster, stronger woman who may not embrace our vision of the female physical 'ideal'. The problem for these women is that they first have to convince society that they have not acquired their muscular physiques through the use of drugs. Because no-one really knows how a highly trained female athlete should look people are often suspicious of a woman who does not conform to our stereotype. Beauty-conscious female American swimmers seem to have a history of narrow-mindedness in this respect. When they were thoroughly beaten by their dedicated East German opponents at the 1976 Montreal Olympics there were the usual complaints about Communist steroid abuse; thankfully, a level-headed section of the American public put their sportswomen in order. Letters to the *New York Times* said:

Perhaps the East German women take their skills more seriously and are capable of viewing themselves as attractive, sexual women, not by their measurements, but because of who they are as human beings.

In contrast to the verbal assault on Eastern countries there is now a growing realisation that the United States has an enormous influence on drug use in sports. At a conference on drug abuse in early 1985, Sir Arthur Gold, President of the European Athletic Association, rebuked other officials for specifically attacking East Germany: 'I ask you to look West to the United States. . . . Much of it [drug abuse] would stop if athletes were not having to keep up with the American Joneses'. Of course, the East Germans are not angels. At Montreal, when comments were made about their masculine physiques and deep voices the East German coach said 'we have come here to swim, not sing'. There are many stories about the organised abuse of steroids by the East Germans. Some of these are probably exaggerated but others have a little more credibility. The 1974 100m breaststroke world record holder was Renate Vogel. When she defected to the West in 1979 she told how steroids were handed around 'along with the vitamin pills'. While official involvement in doping is often attacked as State control by Western critics, and certainly cannot be condoned, there are probably many American or European athletes who would welcome the medical backup that accompanies tacit approval of drug abuse. This is not to say that the East achieves results through its use of doping agents; these female athletes have a reputation for hard work and discipline, something which, until recently, set them apart from women in the West. Dr. Paul Wade is convinced that the fear of 'getting big' prevents our female athletes from stepping over the line into the weights room, yet this is exactly what they must do in order to compete effectively with the Communist bloc women who have more dedication to their sport than to their figures. Resistance to strenuous physical training amongst Western women goes back a long way. Eleanor Holm who won the 100m backstroke event for America at the 1932 Los Angeles Olympics was regarded as a 'Venus of the Waves'. After setting a new Olympic record she probably did a great disservice to the future of women's athletics by saying: 'The moment I find swimming makes me look like an amazon, I'll toss it aside. My appearance is more important to my life as a woman than any championship'. Her lack of commitment became obvious on the 9-day voyage to Germany as part of the 1936 Olympic team. Once on board, her drinking and, for the time, unrestrained behaviour caused a scandal. Before reaching Hamburg she was expelled from the team by members of the American Olympic Committee; despite protestation from the press and some of her fellow athletes she was not reinstated.

Having established the extent of the bias against muscular women in sport it might be possible to approach the question of drug abuse more objectively. Not all 'big' women use anabolic steroids but some certainly do. A spate of disqualifications and bans occurred in the late 1970s as a result of tests for these drugs (see Chapter 1). The first Olympic track and field athlete ever to be disqualified was a woman. Danuta Rosani of Poland qualified for the final of the discus in 1976 but failed the steroid test before having a chance to compete. In 1977 the East German shot-putter Ilona Slupianek lost her gold medal at the European Cup, while Nadyezhda Tkachenko forfeited her pentathlon gold a year later at the Prague-held European Championships. Despite these early warnings, no fewer than seven Olympic class women were banned for life after being caught using steroids in 1979. Part of the reason for these 'scoops' was that the detection methods changed slightly to enable scientists to distinguish between anabolic steroids and the closely related oral contraceptive steroids which had previously interfered with the radiommunoassay stage (see Appendix C).

Although women produce their own androgenic steroids from their adrenal glands, these are not synthesised in amounts large enough to cause masculinising effects. A man taking anabolic steroids is simply adding to his own high levels of anabolic/androgenic hormones and usually looks no more than a bigger, more muscular version of what he was before. Women, on the other hand, by taking anabolic steroids, shift the balance of their appearance so that it resembles that of a

70

man. Their normal menstrual cycle is often suppressed and certain masculine features may appear. For example, the clitoris, which is a penis equivalent, may start to grow (clitoral hypertrophy) to embarassing proportions; the vocal cords may lengthen to deepen the voice and a masculine pattern of hair growth and baldness may begin. All three of these problems are usually irreversible even after the anabolic steroids are discontinued and the inclusion of 'female' hormones (oestrogens) will not prevent their appearance.

Another problem that worries cheating female athletes is the possibility of birth defects as a result of steroid abuse. The foetus is much more susceptible than the adult to the effects of many drugs but anabolic steroids present a unique and frightening problem. Research has shown quite clearly that exposing female animals to androgens, at certain so-called 'critical' periods in their development, can cause masculinisation. In humans the critical period occurs while the baby is still in the uterus and if the pregnant mother is given androgens it can cause a condition in the foetus called 'pseudohermaphroditism' where male sex organs partially develop on an otherwise female body. The danger of giving birth to such babies is very real if high doses of anabolic/androgenic steroids are taken *during* pregnancy. Few women would find themselves in this position since pregnancy usually means a temporary curtailment of competitive athletics.

An interesting, though little mentioned, aspect of anabolic steroid use by women is that of how they affect sexual behaviour. In both male and female primates, including humans, androgens are responsible for sexual urges. In men it is probably testosterone, as the main androgen, that increases the sex drive or libido. In women the production of testosterone is quite low and another androgen, called androstenedione, is also important. This is synthesised by the adrenal gland and is indirectly responsible for the growth of female pubic hair; however it may also influence a woman's sex drive. Studies of women who do not produced adrenal androgens and show reduced libido support this idea[3]. Because of their chemical similarity to androgens, anabolic steroids could increase the sexual appetite of women who take them.

Related to anabolic steroids are oral contraceptive steroids. Many women take these simply to control their menstrual cycles as well as to avoid pregnancy. Should these be regarded as doping agents? There are different types of oral contraceptive but the common 'combined' varieties contain a mixture of synthetic oestrogens and progestagens. The latter is included primarily to build up the lining of the uterus (the endometrium) so that there is some withdrawal bleeding when the month's supply of pills is finished. In this respect the 'period' is an indication that the user is not pregnant and so serves a psychological rather than contraceptive role. The synthetic oestrogens are the main contraceptive component of the combined pill. These suppress the normal hormonal cycle by inhibiting gonadotrophin release from the pituitary (see Figure 3.3) and so prevent the development and release of 'eggs' from the ovary. This ability to interfere with the cycle using drugs allows many women to feel in control of their bodies and hence more confident; in some women the pill can also reduce premenstrual problems like anxiety and water retention, though in others it can exacerbate these difficulties.

Clearly there are many ways in which the female athlete might have an advantage over her non-pill-taking rivals. The main benefit lies in the ability to completely prevent menstruation at the time of competition, but how important a factor is this? At the 1964 Tokyo Olympics only 17 per cent of a sample of 66 sportswomen noted a loss of performance as a result of menstruation; these were usually swimmers. The 1964 and 1968 United States Olympic teams provided more details and it was found that women won gold medals and established new world records at all stages of their cycles; some athletes have given their best ever performances during menstruation[4]. The conclusion that stage of the cycle is unlikely to influence performance will not convince some scientists who believe that women are affected to different degrees. For example, some investigations show that athletic ability varies across the cycle; one of these

72

found that performance in swimming was reduced by about 6 per cent at the time of menstruation[5]. Far more important than the actual period seems to be the premenstrual phase where tension and irritability might affect the athlete's attitude toward competition.

If any effect of menstrual cycle stage on athletic performance could be demonstrated it would probably be the result of endocrine (hormonal) changes. Manipulation of the endocrine system has also been suggested by some experts as being responsible for the diminutive proportions of certain Olympic-class female gymnasts. Dr. Bob Goldman[6] points out that many of the Eastern bloc gymnasts are much smaller for their ages than normal girls; today's top-class female gymnasts might have the physiques of 11 or 12-year-olds up to the age of about 18. The 'Belorussian Bombshell' Olga Korbut was 4 ft 11 in. (1.5m) tall and weighed just 84 lb (38kg) when she thrilled audiences at the 1972 Olympics; most other successful Eastern gymnasts have similar figures. Dr. Goldman believes that those girls might have been given 'brake' drugs to retard their normal development and suggests that a variety of substances could have this effect.

Anabolic steroids can cause a premature sealing of the ends of the growing bones (see Chapter 3) and so have a growth-arresting action. However, it seems unlikely that the masculinising effects of anabolic steroids would go completely unnoticed in petite girl gymnasts. Dr. Goldman has suggested more likely 'brake' drug candidates in the form of LHRH (luteinising hormone releasing hormone) antagonists. LHRH is produced by the hypothalamus and, in women, causes the pituitary gland to release LH and FSH (see Figure 3.3). Without the stimulating effects of LHRH on the pituitary there would be no production of oestrogens or progesterone by the ovaries, thus LHRH antagonists (i.e. substances that oppose the action of LHRH) might be effective in delaying puberty, or even preventing it from ever occurring.

At present there is no evidence that such drugs are being used, and rumours of drug abuse by Communist countries could simply be an angry Western reaction to Eastern bloc success. Many gymnastics coaches believe that such drugs would not even be necessary with strict attention to diet; Bela Karoli, the coach of Romanian gymnast superstar Nadia Comeneci, claims that he is able to keep his girls so small by limiting their fat to less than 8 per cent of their total body weight. Women normally have a fat content of around 22 to 26 per cent; if this drops their normal monthly cycles may become irregular or stop altogether[4], as can happen with menstruating women who train or diet vigorously. Generally speaking, a girl's fat content has to reach about 17 per cent before menstruation will begin; probably Nature's way of preventing pregnancy in semi-starved individuals. Since Karoli ensures his gymnasts have less than half this amount it is not surprising they stay as girls rather than becoming women. Tony Murdoch, secretary of the British Amateur Gymnastics Association (BAGA), is convinced that dieting is the only method currently used by these girls to keep their growth in check:

> They are meticulous in their concern to keep their weight down, so much so that they weigh themselves after every meal. Some of those girls don't have their first period until they're 20.

Mr. Murdoch, along with many other officials, is concerned that doping is not associated with his particular sport and consequently does not see the need for random testing procedures. Perhaps there is no necessity for dope tests in gymnastics, but since the British Sports Council offers its testing services free of charge it simply raises the suspicion of illicit practices if BAGA, and other 'clean' sports, do not take advantage of them.

Although women are closing the gap on men's records they still have a considerable amount of work yet to do. Not surprisingly, to maintain fair play in women's events it has been necessary to introduce sex tests to ensure that successful women are the gender they claim to be. At one time this was done by purely physical examination, the female competitors queuing up in the medical officer's waiting room dressed in only a towel. This procedure was embarassing for officials and competitors alike, so more sophisticated methods were devised. Current sex tests use methods which detect the differences found in cells as a result of having male (XY) or female (XX) chromosomes[7]. Thus, femininity is now determined by demonstrating the existence of the so-called Barr bodies that are present in 20 to 50 per cent of a woman's cell nuclei; men have none at all. This sort of test can be performed on skin cells from inside the mouth (a buccal scrape) or from the root of a hair. The test regulations are described in Appendix B (section 4).

In 1975 Dr. Daniel Hanley, the US representative to the IOC's Medical Committee described sex testing as 'an expensive overreaction to a remote possibility', mainly because a man has never been caught impersonating a woman at the Olympics. This is only true now because of sex tests which, at the time of their introduction, caused a flurry of incidents that more than justified their necessity. At two consecutive Olympic Games the mighty Tamara Press, from Georgia in Russia, dominated the field events. At Rome in 1960 she won the gold medal in the shot put and the silver in the discus; 4 years later at Tokyo she went one better and won the gold in both events. Tamara's sister Irina came sixth in the shot put and it seemed that both women were set to clean-up at Mexico City in 1968. However, when sex-testing was introduced in 1966 the two 'sisters' dropped out of competition, never to return. Exactly the same thing happened with the Romanian world champion high-jumper Iolanda Balas and two more Russians: long-jumper Tatyana Schelkanova and former 400m world record holder Maria Itkina. Whether these athletes were really men or just women dosed with anabolic steroids was never discovered. Another celebrated case is that of Erika Schineggar, the women's downhill ski-racer of 1966. She had her male identity revealed by the advent of chromosome tests in 1967. It was later alleged that 'her' male sex organs had been hidden inside her

75

body since birth. She changed her name to Eric, married a woman and became a father.

In earlier generations, before the advent of the sex test, athletes could be deceptive with more success. The 1946 French European relay silver medallists boasted two members of suspect gender: Claire (later Pierre) Bresolles and Lea (later Leon) Caula both lived life as men after their days in athletics, while the German Olympic high-jumper Dora Ratjen was barred from competition in 1938 when she was found to be a hermaphrodite, having both male and female sexual organs. After she had won the European championships in Vienna with a world record of 5 ft 7 in. (1.7m) the German Athletic Federation said that Ratjen 'had no right to participate in women's competitions'. Dora later became a waiter called Hermann and admitted that he had previously lived the life of a woman for 3 years.

A few years before, track enthusiasts saw intense competition between Helen Stephens (USA) and Stella Walsh (Poland) in the 100m sprint. Stephens was a 6 ft (1.8m), Missouri-born, farm girl who equalled the world record for the 50-yard (45.7m) dash when she was still at high school. Subsequent refinement of her raw power by coach Burton Moore enabled her to beat Walsh, the current Olympic 100m champion, at the 1935 AAU meeting in St. Louis. The reason Walsh was allowed to compete at the national AAU meeting was her dual nationality. She was originally born Stanislawa Walasiewicz in Poland in 1911 but was moved to the USA as an infant where her name was changed. In 1930 she became the first woman to beat the 11 second barrier for 100 yards (91.4m) and Americans thought the Olympic gold was safe. However, she was forced, through redundancy, to take a job at Cleveland Recreation Department which made her ineligible for Olympic competition as someone who earned their living in physical recreation. Consequently, having had no financial help from the USA, she deferred the offer of American naturalisation, took a job with the Polish consulate in New York and ran for Poland in the 1932 Los Angeles Olympics. In winning the 100m gold she probably made enemies, which might explain why she was not granted her naturalisation papers until 1947.

At the Berlin Olympics Helen Stephens produced a tremendous performance and beat Stella Walsh by 2 yards (1.8 m). After the Games a Polish journalist accused Stephens of being a man (despite her being propositioned by Adolf Hitler) and German officials were forced to produce the certification of her femininity. Amazingly, it was Stella Walsh who next hit the headlines after she was shot dead in December 1980 as an innocent bystander at a Cleveland robbery attempt. The autopsy revealed that 'she' had male sex organs; the winner of 41 AAU titles and two Olympic medals was a man[8].

Another Polish sprinter and Olympic medal winner became the subject of controversy in 1967. After the introduction of sex chromosome tests in 1966, Ewa Klobukowska became the first woman to pass a visual examination but fail the genetic test. Her XXY genotype was detected at the 1967 European Cup in Kiev. The six examining doctors said she had: 'one chromosome too many to be declared a woman for the purposes of athletic competition'. She was subsequently stripped of her records and, despite the fact that she was taking oestrogens, banned from competing against women. According to some estimates there are about six 'women' in every 1000 who would not pass a femininity chromosome test. Obviously they live their lives perfectly happily as women yet genetically their sexual status is in doubt. Dr. Renee Richards, the sex-change tennis player, believes the chromosome test is a poor one: 'There are many varieties of patterns and the test is not always a simple XX female or XY male result. There's a whole mosaic of possibilities: XO, XXY, XYY, single X's'. There are also people who suffer from so-called androgen insensitivity syndrome who resemble normal women. This is brought about because they did not respond to male hormones when they were still in the womb. If an athlete clearly has a woman's body why not let her compete as a woman? Surely it should be our physical appearance, not our genetic make-up, that determines our sporting potential.

Suspicions have been raised about the femininity of Jarmila Kratochvilova, the powerful middle-distance runner from Czechoslovakia. She holds world records for the 400m and 800m and won both gold medals at the 1983 World Championships at Helsinki. She was later voted European Sportswoman of the Year. After a long battle to finally beat Marita Koch in 1981, Kratochvilova now dominates the track at major competitions. To Western eyes her gaunt, muscular appearance is far from feminine, but in her quiet village home in Bohemia she claims 'I am just a country girl'. According to her coach Miroslav Kvac this tough upbringing, together with her punishing training programme, is the real secret of her success. Sports journalist Rob Hughes has witnessed her training routine and says:

> the intensity of training is unequalled by any I have witnessed by any other woman and all but a handful of boxers and male athletes in two decades of sports watching[9].

Almost 20 years of Kvac's programme have turned Kratochvilova into a powerhouse of a woman with a motivation to win that matches her strength. She is a certified woman, according to the sex chromosome test, and regards accusations about her gender as ridiculous. Although insinuations concerning advanced hormone substances are rife, particularly amongst disgruntled Western coaches, some people see Kratochvilova's success as the product of training. The American women's Olympic track coach Brooks Johnson insists that his proteges stop regarding Kratochvilova as a freak: 'They have to be willing to train as hard or her accomplishments will never seem attainable.'

The quote that opens this chapter forces us to take sides in the issue of changing female physiques. If we accept that women can never be physically confused with men, no matter how much training they undergo, then we must also accept that 'superwomen' athletes are the product of an artificial process.

Bev Francis is an Australian weightlifter and bodybuilder who weighs nearly 13 stones (85kg) and has a 42 in. (1.2m) chest of solid muscle. Unlike many young women she would not resign herself to a lifetime of dieting; instead she used her natural bulk to best advantage by taking up weightlifting; in her own words she resolved to 'make myself stronger and really achieve something in sport'. She has certainly done that. Bev Francis is probably the strongest woman in the world with squat and deadlift records of over 440 lb (200kg).

Together with other, similarly shaped, women Mrs. Francis has achieved negative results in tests for anabolic steroids but many people are still suspicious of her physique. However, any doubts about the femininity of such athletes could simply be due to a natural bias away from tough, hardworking women. There is no physiological reason to assume that the only way for a woman to become muscular is by abusing male hormones; hard training alone can do it. After all, a woman's breasts, universally accepted symbols of the female gender, are mainly fat, the first thing to go when strenuous exercise burns off excess adiposity. The thick necks and flat chests of these women may stretch the bounds of credibility but perhaps these will become the hallmark of the modern sportswoman.

Western resistance to the physical development of women could seriously hinder the advance of women's athletics such that it never realises its true potential, though hopefully we have now straddled the more difficult social barriers. As more women cross the dividing line between male and female sexual dimorphism the 'he-woman' will achieve more acceptance in a culture which expects women to be nothing but grace and charm.

5

ANTI-ANXIETY DRUGS

In international competition, the difference between two athletes is 20 per cent physical and 80 per cent mental.

Dr. Michael Mahoney,
psychologist at Pennsylvania State University, 1984.

While many sports emphasise the need for physical fitness or
strength, performance in others depends largely on the ability
to *relax*. These include the target sports (e.g. shooting, archery,
darts or golf), certain combat sports (e.g. fencing) and sports
with a danger element (e.g. ski-jumping, bob-sleighing). In
these, the athletes need to stay calm in order to focus their
attention on the skill required. However, many athletes may be
nervous prior to competing owing to the stress and pressures of
the event. As a result of sympathetic nervous activity, they may
have a high pulse rate and may start to tremble or sweat. Hand
tremor will obviously impair performance in sports where fine
motor skills are required. To overcome these feelings, the athlete must learn to relax.

There are many drugs that reduce some of these sympathetic
effects and have been used to reduce anxiety in several sports.
The so-called 'anti-anxiety' drugs, some of which are banned
under current anti-doping legislation, are widely used, but the
extent of their *abuse* is difficult to determine. Is the athlete who
takes a sleeping pill or a glass of beer, to ensure a good night's

sleep before competing, guilty of doping? Or is the athlete who takes a drug to relax *immediately* before an event guilty of doping? These questions have posed several problems for various sporting organisations.

The most commonly used drug is alcohol. This is rapidly absorbed from the stomach and small intestine and quickly distributed around the body. Alcohol can also be absorbed as a vapour through the lungs. It is metabolised in the liver at a rate related to body weight, rather than its concentration, and excreted via the kidneys and lungs. While alcohol affects many tissues such as the stomach, heart, liver, and blood vessels, its effect on the central nervous system is the most noticeable. Contrary to popular belief, alcohol is *not* a stimulant, but a very effective central nervous system depressant and anaesthetic drug. In the higher intellectual centres of the brain there are inhibitory systems that enable us to behave in a restrained and socially acceptable manner. Alcohol *inhibits* these systems and behaviour becomes more spontaneous and less self-critical. By removing these social inhibitions, it appears as if alcohol is having a stimulant effect.

How alcohol affects brain cells is not very clear, but it appears to have a depressant action on the activity of brain cells through a local anaesthetic action. At higher doses the damage may be permanent, since alcohol may act as a *neurotoxin*, and destroy brain cells.

Alcohol intoxication can be divided into four stages. First, the subject feels relaxed with a slight loss of efficiency. In the second, the novice drinker loses all self-control, slurs speech and may not be able to stand, while the hardened drinker speaks and moves with exaggerated care. In the third stage, the subject is unconscious with a flushed face, active sweat glands, red eyes and dilated pupils. In the final stage there is a danger of death from paralysis of the respiratory centre in the medulla (see Figure 2.1).

The effects and after-effects of alcohol intake are well known. Nausea, dehydration, headache, amnesia, impotence and depression are common symptoms of excess intake. The drug is

81

highly addictive, and as tolerance develops, the regular user may become both physically and psychologically dependent. The persistent heavy drinker may become increasingly irritable and eventually develop 'delirium tremens' (the 'DTs') which can induce hallucinations. This condition may even lead to permanent brain damage and death. However, in moderate amounts, alcohol may be used socially for a variety of reasons, to alleviate worry or fatigue or to reduce shyness. The effects experienced often depend on the social situation. Alcohol tends to intensify the existing emotions, while increasing doses of alcohol induce sleep.

Alcohol also impairs skills that are dependent on fine judgement, motor co-ordination or fast reaction times[1]. Thus for many sports, alcohol impairs performance, and most athletes regard excess intake as detrimental to their training programme. In several sports, alcohol is banned by trainers or clubs prior to an event or match. Alcoholic hangovers are known to impair visual acuity, concentration and stamina. Complex skills are more impaired initially by alcohol, although all skills deteriorate as alcohol levels rise. In several countries it is illegal to drive a motor vehicle after drinking alcohol, since it significantly reduces reaction times. The acceptable blood alcohol level varies enormously from country to country, In Denmark the limit is 100mg/100ml; in Norway the limit is 50mg/100ml, while in Britain the limit is 80mg/100ml. This gives some indication of the problems facing sports legislators in fixing levels.

Despite its effects on co-ordination and skills, alcohol is used regularly in certain sports: for example, during darts, snooker, billiards and pool matches which are traditionally organised as a complement to drinking. We are all familiar with players consuming large quantities of alcohol, but still performing superbly in these sports. As a result of national television coverage and sponsorship, usually from the tobacco or alcohol industries, there are often enormous prizes at stake that have elevated these games to professional status. Even so, alcohol has remained as an important aspect of participation. It is difficult to determine to what extent this drinking is for 'effect' or as a true aid to performance.

Under present IOC legislation, alcohol is *not* prohibited. However, blood or breath alcohol levels may be determined at the request of an international federation. This has already been the case at previous Olympic Games in both fencing and shooting competitions. Although fencing is not a sport that particularly lends itself to drug abuse, alcohol has been used to 'steady nerves' before finals with some *apparent* benefits. A limit of 50mg/100ml blood alcohol has been set by the Amateur Fencing Association (AFA) in Britain and dope-testing was introduced for the first time in British fencing at the Martini International Epee Competition held in London in March 1984. The tests were carried out by the Chelsea Drug Centre on four out of eight finalists. The winner and runner-up were tested automatically, and two of the remaining six were chosen by lot. As yet there have been no positive dope tests in British fencing, and according to Raymond Crawford, medical officer of the AFA, doping does not appear to be a problem in either British or international fencing[2].

The 'beneficial' effect of alcohol is unreliable in sustained competitions such as shooting or archery where the need to maintain performance several times a day during 3 or 4 days of competition makes it difficult to control blood alcohol level. Intermittent consumption results in fluctuating alcohol levels and consequently performance is unreliable. While alcohol actually decreases performance at various motor skills, it often increases the drinker's confidence that he is performing better. This increased 'bravado' is an important factor in many 'drink-driving' accidents.

Following bans on excess alcohol in shooting events in modern pentathlon, many competitors in the 1972 Munich Olympics were found to have used other types of anti-anxiety drugs, in particular the so-called minor tranquillisers[3]. The minor tranquillisers include drugs such as meprobamate (Miltown) and the benzodiazepines, e.g. diazepam and chlordiazepoxide (Librium and Valium), that are used clinically to treat anxiety states. Meprobamate blocks the conduction of certain nerve pathways in the brain and spinal cord and acts as a mild tranquilliser without producing drowsiness. However, it is addictive and reduces tolerance to alcohol. The benzodiazepines were originally used as tranquillising agents to reduce aggression in tigers prior to taming them, e.g. for circuses. They act as muscle *relaxants* and, as a result, make one feel less tense and nervous.

While their precise mode of action is not clear, these drugs act on the brain, particularly on parts of the brain using GABA (gamma-amino butyric acid) as their neurotransmitter substance. The benzodiazepines are relatively safe in terms of their low toxicity and they have few side effects. For many years it was thought that they were non-addictive and they were liberally prescribed; suddenly thousands of people were taking anti-anxiety drugs. This fashion was created largely by doctors who were only too happy to have an alternative to the highly addictive barbiturates. Physicians became more wary of the benzodiazepines when it was discovered that patients were becoming dependent on them. After months or years on the drugs, some people experienced severe withdrawal symptoms when they tried to live without them. Depression, acute anxiety attacks, frightening nightmares and hallucinations together with autonomic disturbances were commonly reported. The benzodiazepines remain one of the most useful types of drugs, but their long-term use in treating anxiety is now more carefully monitored.

In contrast to alcohol, the minor tranquillisers could theoretically reduce anxiety without impairing judgement and co-ordination. Therefore in shooting events, the marksman could feel more relaxed and his hand steadier despite the stress of the event. Any side effects of the minor tranquillisers such as headache or drowsiness are only observed after very high doses. Significantly, these drugs are *not* prohibited under current IOC legislation. However, the finding that nearly a *quarter* of all competitors in the pentathlon competition at Munich had used tranquillisers suggested that they were being used extensively as doping agents. Despite many 'red faces' and protests, there were no disqualifications as a result of the tests and it seemed that the marksmen had simply 'progressed' from using alcohol to other types of drugs. More information is needed to determine whether minor tranquillisers do improve performance so that the IOC could decide whether their use constitutes doping. But now that each drug is readily detectable, there is also the possibility that athletes have moved on to other drugs.

In times of stress, one of the most noticeable responses is our rapid heart rate. This response is produced by the release of adrenalin which binds to specific receptor sites on heart tissue. These receptors are known as *beta-receptors*. There are drugs available that can selectively inhibit beta-receptors, known as beta-blockers. They are widely used to treat high blood pressure and certain cardiac disorders such as 'angina pectoris', a pain over the heart brought on by excessive exercise. The beta-blockers include propanolol (Inderal), practolol (Eraldin) and sotalol (Sotacor). These drugs also influence other parts of the sympathetic nervous system and should only be used under careful medical supervision. Recent reports have demonstrated that propanolol can kill sperm, hence their long-term use could result in male infertility[4]. Theoretically, beta-blockers could be used by marksmen to reduce pre-competition tension; but owing to their potentially harmful effects and *possible* use as doping agents, the International Shooting Union placed beta-blockers on its list of banned substances.

Although beta-blockers were not prohibited by the IOC, team doctors at the 1984 Olympics had to fill in declarations for all athletes using beta-blockers and state the doses used. However, this created a loophole for blatant doping in Los Angeles[5]. If competitors produced a doctor's certificate stating that they needed the drugs for health reasons, then they would not be disqualified if drug checks proved positive. However, when urine specimens were screened for these drugs, there were several positives in the modern pentathlon contest. To the amazement of the officials, managers came forward with doctors' certificates covering *whole teams*. When the athletes and teams concerned were not revealed, there was an outcry from both officials and competitors from several countries. In October 1984, the secretary-general of the world body governing modern pentathlon (UIPMB), Colonel Willy Grut, challenged the IOC to reveal the names of the athletes who 'clearly took dope, not for medical reasons, but to improve performance'. He added: 'Just before the contest in Los Angeles, I asked all the team managers at a meeting whether or not any of their athletes had high blood pressure, they all said no'. Colonel Grut was adamant that there should be no cover-up.

It was revealed in November 1984 that the United States and Switzerland had fielded athletes legally on beta-blockers. A report drawn up by Dr. Claus Clausnitzer, of East Germany, on behalf of the IOC's sub-committee on doping and biochemistry in sport, revealed that Peter Minder of Switzerland and Mike Storm of the USA were on beta-blockers and their teams had submitted certificates to that effect. Storm won the individual shooting contest and was fifth overall. This helped the United States team to win the silver team medal. Minder was fifth in the shooting event, enabling Switzerland to come fourth overall. Certain American officials were quick to defend Storm, saying that the medication had been approved by the United States Olympic Committee. According to Ralph Bender, treasurer of the US Modern Pentathlon Association: 'Our team was one of the cleanest there. Nobody must now try to take those silver medals away from us'.

The results embittered many competitors and officials, particularly since it was impossible to determine how many *more* athletes had used beta-blockers. At the Olympics, the first five in the overall competition plus two picked at random were tested. Any number of the remaining 45 athletes may have used the drugs and evaded detection. Moreover, the IOC Medical Commission considered the certificates detailing athletes' complaints as private information, so they were all destroyed after the Games.

One disappointed competitor was Richard Phelps of Britain, who finished fourth in the pentathlon. Phelps had the highest

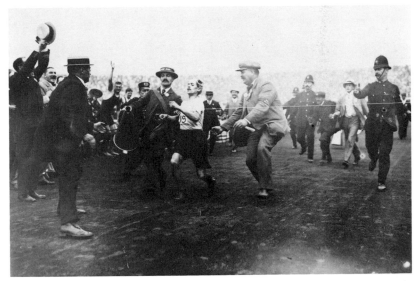

(1) The sensational climax of the 1908 Olympic Marathon in London. Dorando Pietri is helped over the finishing line and subsequently disqualified. Pietri was one of many runners suspected of using the stimulant strychnine.

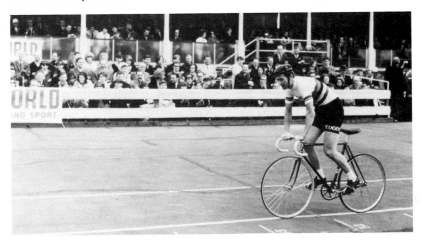

(2) Tommy Simpson, British ex-world professional road-racing champion, died during the 1967 Tour de France after taking amphetamincs.

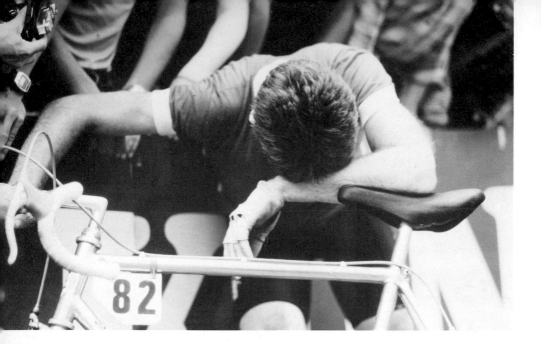

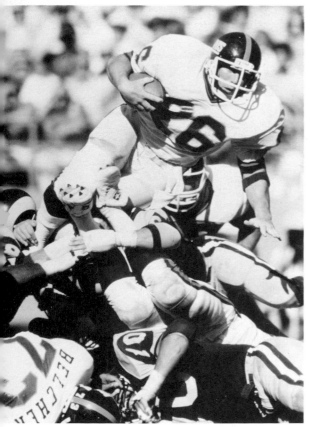

Sean Kelly (above, 3) dominated cycling during 1984, but failed a dope test near the end of the season. Kelly protested his innocence, claiming there had been irregularities in the testing. His appeal was rejected.

The Los Angeles Rams in action (left, 4) against the Raiders. American football is one of the world's most violent sports. It has been alleged that some players try to boost their aggression by using amphetamines, cocaine and anabolic steroids.

Professor Arnold J. Mandell (right, 6) hit the headlines when he exposed the problem of amphetamine abuse by American football players. As team psychiatrist, Mandell was at the centre of a drugs scandal involving the San Diego Chargers.

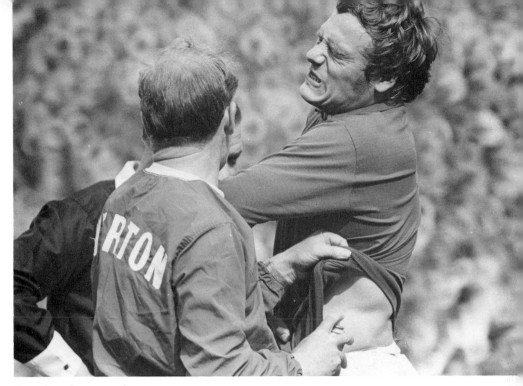

An injured soccer player gets painkilling treatment during a game (above, 5). Painkillers may enable athletes to continue playing but, in so doing, increase the risk of further damage.

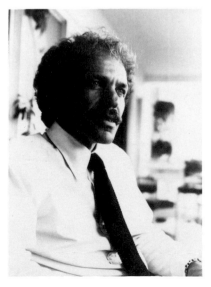

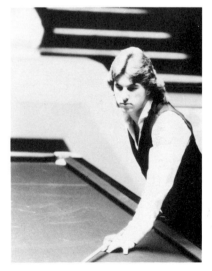

The Canadian snooker player Kirk Stevens (above, 7) was involved in a drugs dispute during April 1985 at the World Professional Championships.

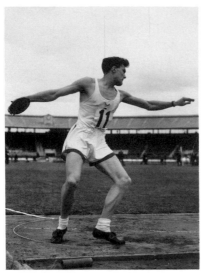

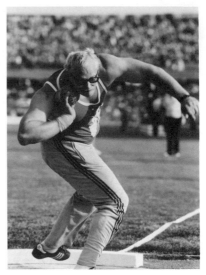

The changing image of male athletes. A discus thrower from the pre-steroid era of the fifties (above, 8). Compare the lean muscular physique of this man with that of the modern athlete.

The modern 'heavy-event' athlete (above, 9). How much are these changes due to diet and training, and how much simply to the use of hormones and anabolic steroids?

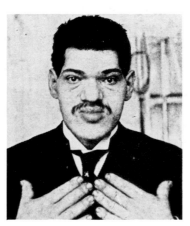

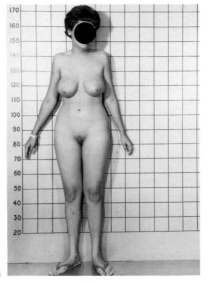

Effective testing for anabolic steroids has forced many athletes to turn to substances such as growth hormones. This may cause 'acromegaly' in which the bones of the face and hands become grossly enlarged (10).

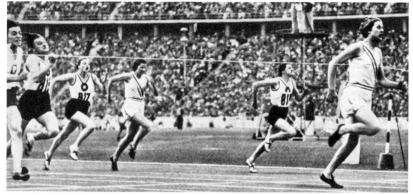

Helen Stephens wins the gold from Stella Walsh (far left) in the women's 100m final at the 1936 Olympic Games (above, 12). After being shot dead at a Cleveland robbery in 1980, Stella Walsh, winner of 41 AAU titles and two Olympic medals, was found to be a man.

The Western media often portray drug abuse in sport as being a problem in Eastern bloc countries. There have been rumours of Russian female gynmasts being given puberty-retarding drugs to create the 'elfin' image typified by Olga Korbut at the 1972 Olympics (right, 13). However, dietary restrictions can produce similar effects.

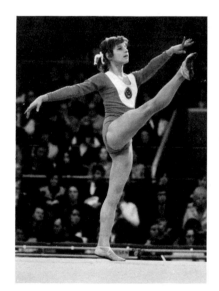

The limitations of examining a person's genetic make-up in sex tests is illustrated by the 'androgen insensitivity syndrome'. This person (left, 11) is genetically *male*, but developed a female body because of insensitivity to male hormones. Under current sex test regulations, this person would not be allowed to compete as a woman!

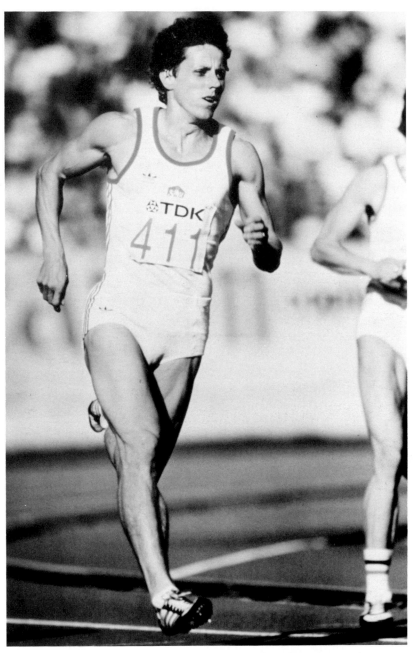

The changing image of female athletes has often prompted accusations
of drug abuse. Many women have developed muscular physiques but

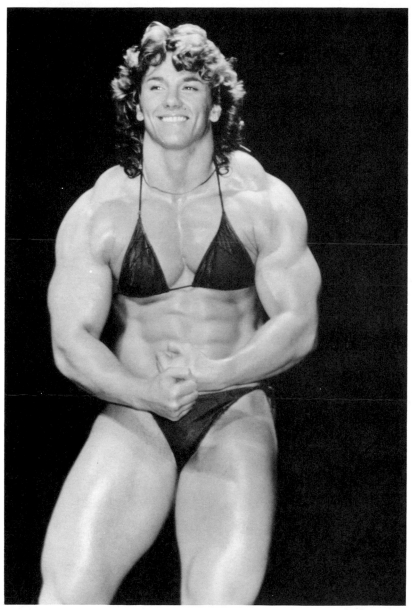

have not failed sex tests or been found guilty of drug abuse. For example, the Czech middle-distance runner, Jarmila Kratochvilova (14), and the Australian body-building champion and weightlifter, Bev Francis (15).

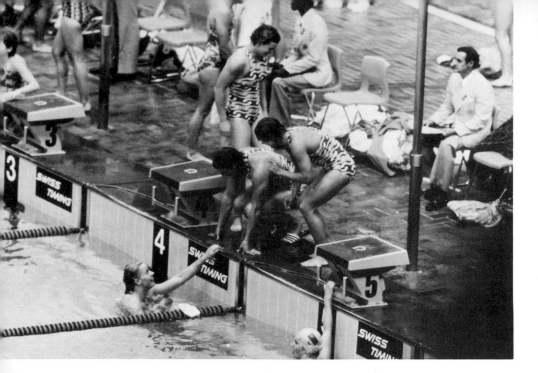

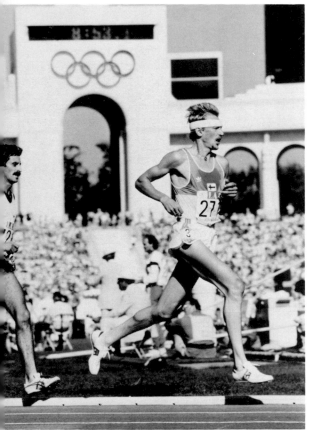

Kornelia Ender is congratulated by her East German team mates at the 1976 Olympic Games in Montreal, in which the East Germans dominated the women's swimming events (above, 16). While there were accusations of steroid abuse, none of the East Germans failed dope tests.

Martti Vainio of Finland (left, 17), silver medallist in the 10,000m at the 1984 Olympic Games, was disqualified after failing a test for anabolic steroids. Vainio was one of several athletes disqualified in Los Angeles for drug abuse.

total score from four events in Los Angeles, but faltered in the shooting. He scored 184 out of 200 on the pistol range. 185 points would have won a bronze medal, 188 points the gold. This illustrates how narrow the margin can be at this level of competition. The incident also fuelled the frustration of those athletes, including Phelps, who were attempting to compete without the help of drugs. The attempt to use 'health reasons' as an excuse amazed many athletes. They could not imagine possible Olympic medallists needing treatment for heart conditions while competing in the pentathlon.

The incident also highlights that if you lose, whatever the reason, then you do not attract publicity or sponsorship. Sponsors are interested in winners, regardless of how rules may be bent or whether drugs were used. The British Modern Pentathlon Association (MPA) is placed in the dilemma whereby if drugs are not used to improve certain aspects of performance, then there is a risk of losing sponsorship. The MPA has two potential champions in Richard Phelps, and Wendy Norman, fourth in the world championships, but are insistent that drug use must be rooted out of the sport. The MPA Honorary Treasurer, Martin Grieves demanded that there should be no cover-up and those who cheat by using drugs should be banned from competition. In a letter to *The Times*, Keith Clark, chairman of the MPA, commented:

> We have been closely involved with drug testing since its inception and in common with a few other governing bodies such as the Amateur Rowing Association, have volunteered for random testing of our athletes throughout the year.

He pointed out that no member of the British team took any banned substance in Los Angeles.

The West German modern pentathlon federation revealed in October 1984 that *six* West German athletes were positively dope-tested at the national championships at Ruhpolding. The West Germans won the team trophy and were sixth at the Los

Angeles Games. The IOC Medical Commission is discussing the problem of beta-blockers in order to introduce stricter control at the 1988 Olympics at Calgary and Seoul. At previous competitions the modern pentathlon officials thought they had already outwitted the cheats by holding the shooting contests on the same day as the cross-country event. In this way, using beta-blockers could be useful in the shooting but would be a disadvantage in the running event. The athlete's answer was to use a beta-blocker with a shorter life, such that it was metabolised before the running event. However, in Los Angeles, there was plenty of time between the events to enable the system to have recovered from the effects of the beta-blockers. Either the legislation or the manner in which the events are conducted need to be changed. One possibility is to combine the running and shooting events as in the Winter biathlon contests; but it is likely that the legislation will have to be stricter not only to cover the use of beta-blockers in modern pentathlon, but also in shooting and archery contests. The legislation may also have to cover other types of anti-anxiety drugs.

Despite their addictive properties, sedative drugs such as barbiturates are still used clinically to relieve tension and anxiety and to induce sleep. These drugs may leave the patient feeling rather drowsy, and again should only be used under medical supervision. Sedatives are not useful as doping agents and are not banned by the IOC.

The nicotine in tobacco smoke can have a rapid calming effect, and many people smoke cigarettes to curb feelings of anxiety. However, any short-term benefits are far outweighed by the risk of bronchitis, lung cancer or heart disease, and the majority of athletes would agree that smoking has a *detrimental* effect on most forms of sporting performance. Smoking causes constriction of the bronchioles in the lungs and carbon monoxide displaces oxygen from red blood cells, resulting in poor breathing and an inefficient oxygen supply to muscles. However, there is a lack of well-controlled studies that have investigated the effects of smoking on sporting performance.

There are also few studies that have examined the effects on performance of smoking marijuana. Marijuana is obtained from the hemp plant *Cannabis sativa*, and the leaves or resin may be smoked or eaten. The drug in its various forms is commonly referred to as 'hashish', 'pot', 'grass' or 'dope'. A 1975 study found no difference between subjects after smoking marijuana and a placebo in terms of vital capacity, expiratory flow and handgrip strength[6]. Mild intoxication with marijuana produces a feeling of relaxation or mild euphoria, so it could be used to reduce pre-competition anxiety.

In August 1980 the French tennis player Yannick Noah was reported to have claimed at the United States Championships that drug-taking was rife among tennis players, and that he found hashish helpful before tournaments[7]. The extent of drug use among tennis players is not known, but it is likely that as rich, young 'jet-setters', at least some players may have experimented with cannabis at some time. (According to Pete Gent, the same is also true for American football players. Gent, a former wide receiver for the Dallas Cowboys, discussed the extent of the problem in his book *North Dallas Forty*.) The International Tennis Federation has not adopted specific legislation regarding drug use other than the following:

> Players shall not at any time within the precincts of a tournament site possess, use, or be under the influence of 'illegal drugs'. 'Illegal drugs' for purposes of this rule are drugs which are illegal under the laws of any place at which an event is being played. Violation of this Section shall result in the player's immediate default from the tournament, a fine up to £5000 and suspension for a period up to ninety days.

Since drugs such as cannabis are illegal in most countries, this would be regarded as an illegal substance under the current legislation. However, drugs that are not illegal under national legislation would therefore be permitted. The International Tennis Federation has recently appointed a medical commission and it is likely the laws regarding drug use in tennis will be re-examined in the near future[8].

While it would be surprising to find that drug use was a problem in cricket, the question was discussed at the Test and County Cricket Board's (TCCB) Spring meeting at Lord's in March 1985. This followed allegations of drug-taking by players on England's 1984 tour of New Zealand and Pakistan. The TCCB were probably also concerned by the amount of publicity given to the case of Ian Botham, the former England captain, who had been found guilty of possessing cannabis. In these cases cannabis was being used as a recreational drug to promote relaxation, rather than as an aid to sporting performance. Nevertheless, the TCCB were concerned about the image of the game and introduced random dope tests from June 1985.

Following recommendations from the Sports Council, the World Professional Billiards and Snooker Association (WPBSA) introduced dope testing in April 1985. The tests began at the World Professional championships in Sheffield and were welcomed by most of the top players. Alex Higgins, the former world champion, said:

> If they feel the need to introduce these tests then so be it. It doesn't really worry me at all. If they want to test me for rabies they are more than welcome. There are enormous pressures on snooker players, but if people are foolish enough to take drugs it won't do their snooker any good.

Less than a week later there were newspaper allegations, based on the claims of the South African player Silvino Francisco, that certain players had been taking drugs. Francisco was alleged to have implicated the Canadian player Kirk Stevens, but later retracted his statements. Mr. Rex Williams, chairman of the WPBSA, said that there was no evidence to substantiate claims that any snooker players had taken drugs. He indicated that should any players be proved to have taken a banned substance, they would be fined both prize money and world ranking points and be banned from the next six tournaments. Second offenders would be banned for life. Francisco was fined 6000 pounds and two world ranking points for bringing the game into disrepute. However Francisco's claim that Stevens was 'as high as a kite' and 'out of his mind on dope' may have had some basis. In June 1985, Kirk Stevens revealed that he was addicted to cocaine and that he had spent around a quarter of a million pounds on the drug during the previous 6 years.

The performance of an athlete is dependent on many factors, for example, motivation, arousal and the ability to control anxiety. Thus for any sport or skill, there is an 'optimum' level of arousal for each individual to reach peak performance. Some competitors may have difficulty getting 'psyched up' for an event due to fatigue, depression, staleness, or having a particular personality type. Alternatively, over arousal may be due to pressures, excessive training or over stimulation with stimulant drugs or 'pep-talks'. Overanxiety, which is more common in introverted personality types, can also lead to impaired performances. This is the main reason for the number of 'false starts' in track-events and is summarised in Figure 5.1 which demonstrates the relation between arousal and performance. The inverted 'U' curve can equally apply to psychological and physical skills. In several sports, over arousal can be reduced by physical exercise, and many athletes report that once the whistle blows or the starting gun is fired, their anxiety disappears. However, in more 'static' events, such as the target sports, this is not the case and the waiting between one shot and the next can make the anxiety worse.

Since there are several problems in separating the social or therapeutic use of anti-anxiety drugs from their doping potential, there is likely to be more controversy in this area in the future. However, athletes can control anxiety without the use of drugs. There are various techniques that can be used, such as progressive relaxation, massage, meditation, biofeedback, yoga or even hypnosis. Mental rehearsal can be useful by imagining the expected stress in advance and constructing ways to cope

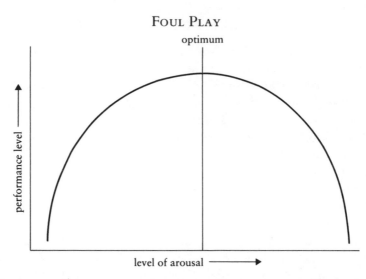

FIGURE 5.1 Graph showing the relationship between performance and arousal. Notice how the level of performance first increases with arousal but, after an optimum level is reached, it starts to drop.

with it. The athlete can 'think through' previous performances and examine previous points of failure and worries from other aspects of life which could impair concentration must be ignored. This psychological preparation not only applies to the 'static' events but also to those where a period of intense concentration precedes a brief, explosive effort such as weightlifting. Indeed for all sports the difference in *psychological* attitude may decide winner and loser in international competition.

6
PAINKILLERS

It is important to remember that these aids deaden a symptom which was originally designed for their protection.

Dr. Vernon Coleman, in Bodypower, *1983*

To succeed in modern sport, athletes are forced to train longer, harder, and earlier in life. They may be rewarded by faster times, better performances and increased fitness, but there is a price to pay for such intense training. These hours of practising the same movements produce gradual wear on specific parts of the body, and while sensible training techniques, footwear and clothes may ease the problem, *overuse* injuries are a serious problem. Constant pressure on young limbs and joints can soon result in damage to tendons, ligaments and muscles. The long-term effects of overuse injuries are not known, but some concerned doctors have asked whether today's gold medallists could be crippled by arthritis by the age of 30. Teenage tennis professionals such as Tracy Austin and Pam Shriver have been plagued by a succession of overuse injuries. Mary Decker ran twice for America at the age of 14, and although she set the indoor record for 880 yards (0.8 km) the following year, she was troubled with injuries for the next 4 years. Decker eventually returned to set seven world records in 1982.

Many athletes are obsessional about training and unwilling to rest despite the pain. Others may be building up to a major event for which they may have already invested months or years of preparatory training. If they are professionals there may be high financial rewards at stake. In each case they might simply ask the doctor or trainer for some type of 'painkiller' or *analgesic* to ease the discomfort and enable them to continue. In addition, there are many injuries that occur during the match or event, particularly in the 'contact' or 'combat' sports. If the injury is not considered to be serious, painkillers may again be administered to enable the athlete to continue. Despite the potential problem of side effects, there tends to be widespread acceptance of painkillers in sport. Most athletes and coaches fail to recognise the damage that can be caused by suppressing pain.

Although we may not always appreciate the fact, pain saves our lives. If something hurts us, we rapidly avoid it and, if wounded, we seek attention. Furthermore, pain may also 'warn' us that we need to rest the damaged area. Pain causes a number of physiological responses such as a sudden intake of breath, vocalisation, a rapid withdrawal from the source of the pain, a drop in blood pressure and a change in the electrical resistance of the skin. There are many types of stimuli that can cause pain, e.g. pressure, heat or a corrosive chemical, and while we clearly perceive each type as painful, the exact mechanism by which this occurs is not known. One possible, though not wholly satisfactory, explanation is that pain is due to excessive stimulation of the sensory systems in the skin responding to heat, cold and touch. Alternatively, there may be specialised 'pain-receptors' in the skin that only respond to tissue damage and are responsible for the sensation of pain. In 1973, Professor Ronald Melzack of McGill University suggested that pain was due to an 'abnormal balance of activity' in the nerves from the skin or from various organs of the body[1]. An important implication of his theory is that it should be possible to reduce pain by stimulation of other parts of the system to restore the balance. The effects of acupuncture may possibly be explained if such stimulation alters the balance of activity that is interpreted as pain. While there is still much to be discovered about how we perceive pain, its crucial *protective* function should be recognised. Moreover drugs that reduce or abolish these 'warning signals' may often be counterproductive.

We are all familiar with the sight of a trainer running on to the pitch during a game to tend an injured player. At one time the trainer would have applied a sponge soaked in ice-cold water to the injured area. More recently, volatile substances are sprayed onto the skin from an aerosol can. In both cases the rapid cooling of the skin produces temporary relief, but such treatment is obviously very limited. There are a number of drugs that may be administered to injuries prior to the game that have prolonged effects. These *local* anaesthetic agents include drugs such as procaine (Novocain), lidocaine (Xylocaine) and bupivacaine (Marcaine). Injections of local anaesthetic drugs can produce cardiac disorders and should not be used 'on the field'. In very large doses they cause central nervous system stimulation, convulsions and death[2]. The IOC permits the use of local anaesthetics only where there is medical justification and only with the aim of enabling the athlete to continue competing. If local anaesthetics have been used, the IOC Medical Commission has to be notified at least 24 hours before the competition[3].

When body tissue is damaged, substances called *prostaglandins* are synthesised and released as part of an inflammatory response. This consists of dilation of local blood vessels producing redness, fluid release producing swelling and nerve endings are sensitised, resulting in increased pain. However, there are a number of so-called 'anti-inflammatory' drugs that are not banned by the IOC. These are used to treat a wide range of aches and pains, rheumatism and arthritis. The most common anti-inflammatory drug is acetylsalicylic acid, better known as aspirin. Aspirin blocks the synthesis of prostaglandins and thus prevents the anti-inflammatory response. It is cheap, very effective and quite safe, although prolonged use with high doses can cause gastrointestinal irritation as well as effects on the central nervous system. Also, since intra-uterine devices (IUDs) are partially dependent on prostaglandin release for their contraceptive effectiveness, the continued use of aspirin-type drugs increases the risk of pregnancy in women using IUDs as a form of contraception[4].

Other anti-inflammatory drugs include naproxen, indomethacin (Indocin), oxyphenbutazone (Tanderil) and phenylbutazone (Butazolidin) commonly known as 'bute'. These drugs are more powerful than aspirin but their side-effects are often more serious. (An exception is the drug ibuprofen which is quite powerful but appears to have fewer side effects.) Their prolonged use may lead to gastrointestinal effects such as ulceration or perforation of the stomach or intestines, and diarrhoea is a commonly reported side effect. In addition to effects on the liver and blood cells, they affect the central nervous system causing headaches, dizziness or disorientation. Phenylbutazone can cause fluid retention, and is therefore unsuitable for female athletes who already suffer from pre-menstrual fluid retention. Due to the number of possible adverse reactions, these drugs should only be used under careful medical supervision. However, 'bute' is used as much as, if not more than, aspirin by some athletes, such as American footballers, to reduce pain and swelling in joints and ligaments.

A Washington consumer group recently called for bans on both phenylbutazone and oxyphenbutazone on the grounds that they believed their side effects may have led to 10,000 deaths worldwide[5]. One official from an American company that markets phenylbutazone was reported as saying that it had been supplied to 180 *million* patients since 1952. Since then he claimed there had been 1200 deaths, but it was not certain whether these were due to direct effects of the drug. Both drugs have been available on prescription in Britain since 1964. In December 1983 the Minister for Health, Kenneth Clarke, in a letter to the House of Commons, said that there had been 1685 reported cases of adverse reactions to Butazolidin including 442 deaths in Britain, and 503 reports of suspected adverse reactions to Tanderil, including 131 deaths. In August 1984 the British Committee on Safety of Medicines decided that oxyphenbutazone should be withdrawn from routine use. It is permitted for the treatment of arthritis in hospitals under careful supervision.

In America, the Food and Drugs Administration is currently reviewing the use of similiar painkillers. In some states in America, 'bute' is already forbidden for use in racehorses by the racing commissions, because the effects are unpredictable. Horses with sore knees may apparently run better following treatment with bute, but sometimes their knees 'give way' unexpectedly.

For *prolonged* pain-relief, athletes use other types of drugs, in particular the *corticosteroids*. During times of stress the cortico-steroids are produced by the cortex of the adrenal glands (see Figure 6.1). Their release is under the influence of a substance released from the pituitary gland called adrenocorticotrophic hormone (ACTH). The adrenal cortex is essential to life, and if removed, death will occur within days. Corticosteroids can be classified into two groups: the glucocorticoids and the minera-locorticoids. Glucocorticoids (cortisol, hydrocortisone, corti-costerone) act to suppress inflammation, promote the use of fatty acids for energy and accelerate the formation of glucose from protein. Mineralocorticoids (e.g. aldosterone) control salt and water balance by acting on the tubules in the kidneys to promote the retention of sodium and water.

These steroids are commonly used in the treatment of arthri-tis and soft tissue injuries. These drugs act by suppressing the inflammatory response of the tissues to injury. They can be delivered precisely to the injured area by injecting into the joint with a local anaesthetic. The corticosteroids are available in various commercial preparations such as betamethasone, dexa-methasone (Decadron) or methylprednisolone, and are widely used to treat overuse injuries such as 'tennis elbow'.

In the same way as using sympathomimetic amines, some athletes, particularly racing cyclists, have used corticosteroids to mimic the effects of sympathetic nervous activation. Corti-costeroid treatment can produce feelings of well-being or even euphoria. These substances may act as both stimulants and painkillers, but their prolonged administration in large doses produces serious physical side effects as well as psychotic reac-tions. The retention of sodium and water leads to cardiovascular

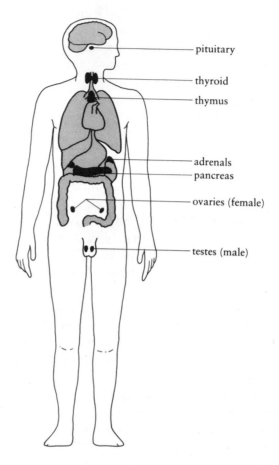

pituitary

thyroid

thymus

adrenals

pancreas

ovaries (female)

testes (male)

FIGURE 6.1 The location of the various hormone-producing (endocrine) glands.

problems and laying down of excess fat. They can also cause increased susceptibility to infection (e.g. skin disorders such as acne). In women, there may also be menstrual disturbances and abnormal hairiness.

In general, patients withdrawn from corticosteroids cannot cope with physical stressors such as infection or injury. Treatment with corticosteroids may suppress the secretion of ACTH and so the adrenal cortex degenerates. Therefore, once the treatment stops, the recipient may suddenly suffer from adrenal *insufficiency*. This occurs naturally in the condition known as Addison's disease. The condition results in cardiovascular problems due to the decreased blood volume and the consequent increase in blood viscosity. If athletes are taking corticosteroids, they may have to be slowly 'weaned off' over a period of months. Other athletes may be using ACTH to stimulate corticosteroid release, so that only endogenous, and therefore non-detectable, corticosteroids are released.

The IOC has condemned the use of corticosteroids, and is currently testing for excess ACTH levels. The 'normal' range of corticosteroid concentrations varies considerably from person to person; therefore, any quantitative measures are difficult to enforce. One famous incident from the horse racing world highlighted the problem. In 1967 the racehorse Hill House won the Schweppes Gold Cup at Newbury, but a dope test revealed abnormally high levels of steroids in the urine. Further tests revealed that the horses's 'normal' levels of corticosteroids were far higher than other horses, which eventually satisfied the racing authorities[6]. However, there are many cases of athletes artificially manipulating their levels of corticosteroids. For example, there have been several racing cyclists who have suffered illnesses directly related to prolonged use of corticosteroids. In November 1978 the Tour de France winner, Bernard Thevenet, admitted he had 'ruined his health' as a result of their use.

The extent of current corticosteroid or ACTH use among athletes is not known, but according to reports from America, cortisone is frequently used by both football and basketball players, although about only one-tenth as often as bute. There was some controversy at the 1980 World Championships when it was discovered that Rosa Colorado of Spain, winner of the 400m hurdles race, had an injection containing steroids to help heal a broken finger[7]. As with testosterone, it is difficult for officials to distinguish between naturally occurring, endogenous corticosteroids and those that have been injected. Cortisone creams *are* permitted to treat eczema and allergic skin reactions.

In addition to local anaesthetics and anti-inflammatory drugs, pain can be alleviated by various drugs which act *centrally* without producing general anaesthesia. The best known are morphine, its derivatives and similar synthetic substances called the *narcotic analgesics*. Natural opiates come from the seed pod of the Oriental poppy (*Papaver somniferum*). They have been used for hundreds of years to induce sleep, relieve pain and produce altered states of consciousness. In 1805 a German chemist managed to isolate the active ingredient from opium and called it morphine after Morpheus, the Greek god of dreams. Seventy years later diacetlymorphine or *heroin* was produced. Both substances were used to treat severe pain.

Morphine is readily absorbed when smoked, eaten or injected. Its effects are seen after about 30 minutes and may last for up to 12 hours. Morphine acts on the cerebral cortex to reduce fear, anxiety and pain, and generally produces a feeling of well-being. The analgesic effects of morphine are mediated via an area in the brain called the periaqueductal grey region. While morphine can have an initial powerful stimulant effect, it also acts on the cerebellum resulting in poor motor co-ordination (see Figure 2.1). It has both excitatory and inhibitory effects on centres in the medulla. Low doses of morphine stimulate the 'vomiting centre' and associated centres to produce other symptoms such as sweating. It also stimulates the 'vagal centre' to produce lowered pulse rate, but in high doses depresses the respiratory centre in the medulla. Thus, large doses kill the recipient by stopping respiration. Other centrally mediated effects include dry mouth, itching, lethargy and loss of appetite. Tolerance to morphine develops rapidly, and within 2 to 3 weeks, larger doses are needed to produce the same effect. Since the withdrawal symptoms are so unpleasant, the user eventually becomes addicted to the drug. Heroin is far more powerful than morphine, and is only used clinically to treat severe pain.

The use of narcotic analgesics is strictly controlled in most countries, with unlicensed possession classified as a criminal offence carrying harsh penalties. However, drugs such as heroin are widely abused for their psychological effects, and there is a disturbing acceleration in the number of heroin addicts in Britain and America, particularly among the teenage population.

The use of narcotics in sport is rather surprising considering some of their known effects. However, heroin was used by boxers for its anaesthetic and stimulant properties. In 1963 the New York welterweight Billy Bello died of heroin poisoning. There is also a long history of morphine injections being used by cyclists for its initial powerful stimulant effect. During the latter phase of a race, cyclists could inject themselves to achieve the 'final kick' for the finishing sprint and then immediately relax after the race due to the sedative effect of the drug. The IOC has banned the use of *all* narcotic analgesics (see Table 6.1), but permits certain anti-inflammatory drugs and non-narcotic analgesics for the relief of pain.

TABLE 6.1   Examples of narcotic analgesics currently banned by the IOC

Anileridine	Morphine
Codeine	Oxocodone
Dextromoramide	Oxomorphone
Dihydrocodeine	Pentazocine
Dipipanone	Pethidine
Ethylmorphine	Phenazocine
Heroin	Piminodine
Hydrocodone	Thebacon
Hydromorphone	Trimeperidine
Levorphanol	and related compounds
Methadone	

Many team doctors have wanted to use *codeine* as an analgesic. Its effects are weaker than those of morphine, there are fewer side effects, it does not affect respiration and it is not as addictive. Codeine is already a widely used component of simple analgesics and as tablets of codeine phosphate is useful in the treatment of traveller's diarrhoea. The problem is that codeine, like morphine, is an opiate. It is difficult to distinguish from other opiates because it is metabolised in a similar fashion to morphine. Thus, codeine is regarded as a doping agent by the IOC.

In the 1976 Winter Olympics in Innsbruck, the captain of the Czechoslovakian ice-hockey team, Frantisek Pospisil, was disqualified when a urine test revealed traces of codeine. Both the points and the goals that Czechoslovakia had accumulated against Poland in a previous game were annulled, and the team doctor was reprimanded. The International Ice Hockey Federation protested to the IOC regarding the decision, and the President, Dr. Sabetzi, complained that the decision was 'unjust'. There had been a 5 to 4 vote in favour of the decision at the IOC Medical Commission. Pospisil was unhappy since he claimed he had simply taken the treatment to combat influenza. Surprisingly, the IAAF regulations specifically *permits* the therapeutic use of codeine, but the problem remains in deciding whether an athlete has used the drug therapeutically or as a doping agent.

Recent research has revealed why the opiates are so effective in relieving pain, and have also caused one of the most exciting developments in brain research. It has been shown that the brain produces its own substances that act like morphine. These naturally occurring or endogenous substances have been called the *endorphins*. When these substances are released, they bind to specific receptor sites in the central nervous system to produce their effects. Regions associated with 'pain pathways' in the brain and spinal cord are rich in these receptor sites, so morphine and other narcotics may simply be mimicking the action of these naturally occurring endorphins by binding to their receptor sites. Since their discovery in the mid-1970s, chemists have managed to isolate and identify these so-called 'endogenous opiates'. There appear to be at least two different types, both composed of amino acids, the building blocks of proteins. One type is called beta-endorphin which is secreted into the bloodstream by the pituitary gland, and acts like a hormone. The other type are much smaller and have been called the 'enkephalins', which means 'in the head'. These substances may act more locally, perhaps as a neurotransmitter (see Chapter 2).

One popular theory suggests that these chemicals are released during periods of either physical or psychological stress. It is known that the level of endorphins increases during strenuous exercise. The exercise-induced release of endorphins probably contributes to the menstrual disturbances that many women athletes report following regular, strenuous exercise[8]. Like exogenous opiates, they mask the pain of exercise and it has been suggested that endorphin release produces the psychological 'high' or 'peak experience' that many athletes report during a good run. Perhaps endorphins are also produced during sexual activity to produce feelings of contentment or well-being. Furthermore, it has been argued that some runners become *addicted* to the endorphins released during exercise, i.e. they are 'hooked' on a substance produced by their brain.

While this is an intriguing possibility, a recent study by Robert McMurray and his colleagues at the University of North Carolina at Chapel Hill raises some doubts. In their 1984 study they injected volunteers with either a 'control' substance or with *naloxone*, a drug that blocks the action of the endorphins[9]. Naloxone is used clinically to treat patients who have taken an opiate overdose. The volunteers walked on a treadmill that gradually became steeper and more difficult to walk on. They were asked to stay on the treadmill as long as possible and describe at intervals how they felt. There was no difference between the naloxone and control group in terms of time taken to reach exhaustion or perceived exertion. None of the subjects reported feeling anything other than exhaustion during and directly after the exercise. Therefore it appeared that endorphins were not involved. McMurray suggested that the 'high' or feeling of well-being could simply be due to the release of built-up stress or due to the effects of adrenalin.

The analgesic effects of acupuncture can be blocked by naloxone, but when pain is reduced by hypnotic suggestion, naloxone has no effect. Thus acupuncture, but not hypnosis, appears to cause the release of endorphins. Pain can successfully be reduced in some patients by administering a placebo or pharmacologically inert substance. This pain reduction seems to be mediated by endorphins because it is blocked by naloxone, i.e. when patients take a pill that they think will reduce pain, it does so *pharmacologically* by triggering the release of endorphins[10].

In recent years there has been an increase in 'jogging' as a means of getting fit. Since many joggers run with music playing via portable tape recorders, it is interesting to note a study recently reported in the journal *Psychology Today*[11]. At the Ohio State University, Drs. Miller and Tejwani tested experienced runners on two treadmill trials, either with or without music playing through earphones. Although the amount of exercise was the same for each trial, all the runners reported that the running was easier *with* the music playing. While heart rates were similar, the endorphin levels of the runners listening to the music increased, but not as much as in those who ran without the music. Therefore music reduced the exercise-induced release of endorphins. Miller suggested that fewer endorphins were produced because the runners felt that the exercise was easier with music playing. Thus the body's biochemistry is affected by the psychological perception of the stress. This point raises several questions about our understanding and our *attitude* to pain.

There are numerous reports of soldiers in combat or athletes during competitions who did not realise that they were seriously injured until the event was over. In soccer, Bert Trautmann, the Manchester City goalkeeper, broke his neck during the 1956 FA Cup Final against Birmingham City. Manchester City won the game, and Trautmann did not realise the extent of his injuries until after the end of the match. While it is possible that the release of endorphins could mask the pain, it appears that during times of stress the brain apparently 'ignores' certain pain signals. Interviews with arrivals at hospital casualty wards indicate that many do not feel very much pain following injury. The pain is somehow being suppressed in these cases. Contrary to what we might predict, there does not always seem to be a direct relation between the extent of injury and the pain experienced. A small cut or burn can be very painful immediately, while serious damage, for example from a gunshot wound, may not be painful for some time later. How does the brain 'decide' when and what to perceive as painful?

The traditional view of how we perceive pain was described by René Descartes 300 years ago. He argued that if, for example, we stepped on a flame, a message was rapidly passed from the foot to the brain via the spinal cord, and the brain returned a message that told the foot to move quickly. This seems reasonable until we examine what can happen in practice. Patients can experience pain even when there is nothing physically there to register it, e.g. following amputation of a limb.

There is no doubt that mental processes affect physiological processes, and vice-versa, but how this occurs with respect to pain is not clear. We all have different pain 'thresholds', and the personality, attitude and past experiences of any individual will determine how he or she responds to pain. Some of the most interesting research in this area has been conducted by Patrick Wall, Professor of Anatomy at University College, London. He has presented his 'gate-control' theory to explain how the brain recognises pain[12]. Stimulation of certain pathways can prevent pain signals being detected by the brain. On the practical side, Wall's research has led to advances in the clinical management of pain, using alternative methods to drugs. In some remarkable studies, pain relief was achieved by electrical stimulation of 'inhibiting nerves' at the site of the wound. By activating this 'inhibiting' system that has ceased to function in the damaged area, patients have been able to 'switch off' pain using an electrical stimulating device, although the techniques are still very much in their infancy. Professor Wall recognises the protective function of pain but suggests that pain control can be 'overdone'.

To succeed in many sports, athletes have to overcome the 'pain barrier', and the 'courage' and 'strength' of the exhausted marathon runners are often admired by spectators. Unfortunately, the careers of many young athletes have ended prematurely either as a result of psychological pressures or from a succession of overuse injuries. In many cases the warning signals were ignored until it was too late. Pain signals are acting to prevent over exertion, permanent injury or even death. It is dangerous to suppress or abolish these signals with drugs simply to enable an athlete to compete.

7

CURRENT TRENDS

At least 80 per cent of top sportsmen are slaves of hormone products.

Paul Nevala, Finland's former Olympic javelin champion,
March 1981.

The possible dangers and penalties involved has not prevented doping in sport, and when the consequences have been *fatal*, many athletes have continued to use drugs. Following Tommy Simpson's death in 1967, the Belgian cyclist Roger de Wilde and the Spaniard Valentin Uriona both died after taking amphetamines. Amphetamines were also thought to have played a part in the death of a league soccer player in Greece in 1973[1]. Since then dope testing has forced athletes to switch to 'undetectable' drugs, and it is likely that there are now more substances being used as doping agents than ever before. In November 1983 the international shot-putter, Mike Winch, a member of the International Athletes Club, pleaded for more severe action by authorities on the use of drugs in sport. He argued that the use of drugs was accelerating and becoming increasingly dangerous[2].

Since most stimulants are now readily detectable, the use of other substances has increased dramatically. In his 1980 book on Eastern drugs, Dr. Stephen Fulder describes a substance used regularly by Soviet athletes as a stamina-building drug[3]. It is a substance that does not fit into any of the IOC banned drug categories, and despite extensive use in the Soviet Union over the last 20 years, little is known about it in the West. It is an extract of the thorny creeping plant called *Eleutherococcus senticosus*, which belongs to the family Araliaceae, the same family as ginseng. The plant grows wild in Siberian forests, and is known to increase stamina and performance, but does not have the side effects of the classical stimulant drugs.

Its properties were originally discovered in a screening programme directed by Professor Brekhman at the Vladivostok Laboratory of the USSR Academy of Sciences. An early trial reported that runners in a 10km race were, on average, 5 minutes faster after *Eleutherococcus* treatment than runners receiving a placebo treatment. The reported increase in endurance was confirmed by Professor Korobkov at the Lesgraft Institute of Physical Culture and Sport in Moscow, in large trials involving 1500 athletes. The only side effect reported was an occasional transient rise in blood pressure.

Eleutherococcus is widely used in Russia as a general 'tonic' by people performing tasks requiring prolonged concentration or involving stress, ranging from deep sea divers to assembly-line workers. Since it does not impair judgement, it has also been used by lorry drivers and pilots. The Russian cosmonauts, Vladimir Lyakhov and Valery Ryumin, were reported to have taken some every morning during their 185-day record-breaking stay in space in the Salyut 6-Soyuz 32 space station. In laboratory experiments, *Eleutherococcus* was found to increase the time that mice could swim until exhaustion by up to *44 per cent*. Human studies also suggested that *Eleutherococcus* treatment could increase stamina, co-ordination, and concentration.

The Russians went on to investigate several other 'anti-fatigue' substances from various plants as well as other traditional Eastern medicinal substances such as pantocrine and schizandra. The common link in each case was that the active components were *glycosides*[4]. According to Dr. Fulder, these particular glycosides act directly on the hypothalamus which in turn influences the output of the adrenal glands, through the release of ACTH (see Chapter 6). Hence, Dr. Fulder claims that

Eleutherococcus can reduce the stress response, and whether the subjects are laboratory animals, hospital patients or factory workers, the benefits cannot be disputed.

Since *Eleutherococcus* is widely used as a general tonic, athletes could argue that it was not being used specifically to improve performance. Research has suggested that it is most effective if it is taken on a daily basis between 10 days and a month prior to the event. In 1974, Professor Korobkov wrote that *Eleutherococcus* and similar substances have

> nothing in common with doping, their action is primarily aimed at accelerating the restorative processes after intensive activity and at increasing the body's resistance to unfavourable external influence.

It was reported to be useful for endurance events such as boxing, long-distance running and swimming, rather than the 'explosive' sports such as weightlifting or sprinting.

Eleutherococcus does not fit into any of the IOC's banned drug categories in terms of either chemistry or effects. Hence it is legal as far as Olympic athletes are concerned. Even if the IOC decided to ban *Eleutherococcus*, it would be difficult to enforce, since it is reported to be effective even if the course of treatment stops before the contest.

Despite the claim that *Eleutherococcus* is used as a tonic, the plant has stamina-building properties; should it therefore be regarded as a doping agent? If so, then the same would have to apply to other herbal 'tonics' or 'stimulants'. For example, according to Ancient Chinese medicine, the extract of ginseng root has many properties including the reduction of fatigue during exercise. One study reported that rats treated with ginseng had less muscle glycogen depletion during prolonged swimming than control animals, but no differences were found in swimming endurance[5]. Surprisingly, there are very few scientific studies that have investigated the effects of 'herbal' stimulants on sporting performance.

The examples of *Eleutherococcus*, ginseng or related substances raises important questions about the definition of a drug. *Any* substance that interacts with and influences a biological system must be regarded as a drug. This applies equally to naturally occurring or synthetic products. In earlier times, drugs tended to be extracts from plants, that had been found by practical experience to have certain physiological or psychological effects, e.g. smoking, chewing or swallowing the leaves, roots or seeds. It was only relatively recently that 'pure' drugs were isolated and chemicals with similar properties synthesised, and it is simply for historical reasons that many of the prohibited drugs are synthetic substances. The newer 'mild stimulants' such as pemoline or centrophenoxine are synthetic compounds, while cocaine and caffeine are naturally occurring substances, but all are now regarded as doping agents.

Dichloracetic acid is a drug that could theoretically enhance endurance by indirectly decreasing the production of lactic acid. Lactic acid build-up is partially responsible for the cramp-like pain in the side, commonly known as 'stitch'. According to a 1981 report, rats treated with dichloracetic acid had swimming times that were *40 per cent* longer than control animals in an endurance test. The effect was apparently due to a slower accumulation of lactic acid in muscle and blood of the drug-treated rats[6]. It is not currently known whether dichloracetic acid enhances sporting performance, or whether it has significant side effects. Since it is the build-up of acid that contributes to fatigue in many types of exercise, it would seem reasonable to assume that ingesting an 'alkalinising buffer' solution prior to exercise might delay the onset of fatigue. According to Professor David Lamb, contradictory findings have been reported. In one study, raising the pH of the body fluids by ingesting sodium bicarbonate increased cycling endurance, while another[7] found no effect of 'buffering' on the time taken to sprint 400m. It is unlikely that sodium bicarbonate would be useful as a doping agent since large doses can cause vomiting and diarrhoea.

The anorectic properties of stimulant drugs were exploited by certain sportsmen to get down to the appropriate weight for their sport. Now that these drugs are detectable, other substances have been used. Diuretic drugs have been taken to lose weight and enable athletes to participate in lower weight categories. These drugs, which increase urine flow, are used clinically to eliminate water from body tissues in certain pathological conditions, or to remove the bloated feeling that some women experience as a result of pre-menstrual fluid retention. After having been weighed, the athlete can then drink a large amount of fluid to replace the water lost, or infuse liquids intravenously. Owing to the dramatic disturbances in electrolyte balance, this practise is extremely dangerous in terms of effects on the heart and kidneys. The IOC Medical Commission has suggested to the International Sports Federations that competitors should be weighed before and after competition, and examined for any evidence of intravenous infusion[8]. The use of diuretic drugs is not recommended as a means of weight loss. It is simply body *fluid*, not fat, that is removed and which has to be replaced. Chemicals to induce vomiting or diarrhoea have also been used by athletes to cause weight loss. This abuse not only causes dehydration, but also excessive potassium loss resulting in muscle weakness.

Athletes have used other substances to lose weight rapidly. In 1980, Muhammed Ali, a leading campaigner against the use of drugs, admitted that he took a *thyroid* drug prior to his world heavyweight title fight with Larry Holmes[9]. Ali had been out of action for 2 years, and he used the drug to get his weight down. Thyroid overactivity does produce a general loss of weight by decreasing fat and carbohydrate reserves and increasing urine flow. Metabolic rate is increased, and typical symptoms include staring eyes, often with protrusion of the eyeballs, because fat has been deposited behind them. It is possible that using a thyroid drug may then inhibit normal thyroid function and produce a period of relative thyroid *deficiency*. This is characterised by lowered metabolic rate, slow pulse and impaired mental functions. Ali lost the fight to Holmes, and while there are obviously several alternative explanations, it is feasible that the after-effects of the drug may have impaired his performance.

111

Anabolic steroids are still used by athletes at international competitions. Several athletes were disqualified for using steroids at the 1984 Olympic Games, including silver medallists Vainio and Johansson, the weightlifters, Tahra and Tarbi and the Greek javelin champion Anna Verouli. Two Canadian weightlifters, Hadlow and Chagnon, were both sent home when urine samples obtained during training periods 2 weeks before the start of the Games were found to contain methyl-testosterone. During the same week the American weightlifter Jeff Michaels failed in a last-ditch attempt to compete in Los Angeles. He had been one of the weightlifters disqualified at the 1983 Pan-American Games in Caracas, but had personally appealed against the 2-year ban from competition on the grounds that the testing procedures were invalid. Had Michaels competed, he would certainly have been favourite for the super-heavyweight gold medal. However, it is the Canadian weightlifters who are building a reputation for drug use. In 1983 three Canadian weightlifters were arrested at Montreal airport on their way back from an international event when *22,000* anabolic steroid tablets were found in their luggage.

The disqualifications in Los Angeles were not confined to the athletes. The Japanese masseur, Yoshitaka Yahagi was disqualified and banned from the 1988 and 1992 Games for giving a drug to a competitor and telling him that it was a herbal product. According to the IOC, Yahagi gave Mikiyashu Tanaka, a member of the volleyball team, a compound that contained several prohibited substances to clear a cold. Tanaka was allowed to continue in the Games. Several cases of doping were not revealed until some months after the Olympic Games. For example, in September 1984 two Norwegian Olympic oarsmen were suspended by their national sports federation for breaking doping regulations. Espen Thorsen and Vetle Vinje, members of the team which finished eighth in the quadruple sculls at Los Angeles, were tested in Norway on June 29th, more than a month before the Olympic finals and excessive amounts of testosterone were found[10]. Since 'excess' testosterone is measured by comparing levels of epitestosterone with

112

testosterone, it is possible that athletes might try to avoid detection by injecting epitestosterone to balance the ratio.

A new threat emerged in 1983 when it was revealed that athletes at events in Helsinki were using a growth hormone to enhance size and strength. None of the 200 samples taken were positive for steroids, but according to a *Los Angeles Times* report, the IOC Medical Commission found traces of growth hormone in the urine samples tested at the Cologne laboratories. No athletes were disqualified, because it is not on the banned list of substances. Growth hormone or somatotrophin is believed to enhance body size and strength *more* effectively than anabolic steroids or testosterone, and is thought to have fewer side-effects[11]. Dr. Robert Kerr, who has prescribed somatotrophin to American athletes for 3 years, describes it as 'an elite drug in track and field competition today'. Kerr claims that the top athletes are using somatotrophin in preference to anabolic steroids, and that the effects are more lasting. Kerr argues that if an athlete stops taking steroids he will lose a percentage of the gains in strength and size, but with somatotrophin the gains tend to stay. Prince Alexandre de Merode, chairman of the IOC Medical Commission, told the *Los Angeles Times* that IOC doctors have been investigating the use of somatotrophin for several months, but as yet there are no *reliable* testing methods. Since somatotrophin is not officially banned by the IOC, it has been suggested that athletes, particularly in the United States, are using it extensively and it remained technically 'legal' in the Los Angeles Olympics.

Whether somatotrophin affects performance is not certain, but it does promote growth and is prescribed for children with stunted growth, whose pituitary glands do not produce enough of the substance. It is very expensive because it has to be extracted from the pituitary glands of human corpses, a process which had led it to be dubbed the 'dead man's drug'. Unfortunately, it is in short supply for treating children with growth problems, yet athletes are using it extensively to increase size. It is a sad testimony to the continuing determination of some athletes, coaches and a few unscrupulous doctors to beat dope controls that a large black market trade in somatotrophin has developed. In December 1983 Neil Macfarlane, speaking in the House of Commons, named a British drug runner who is at present earning a black market income from a base in France. His 'drugs-by-post' service to athletes includes steroids and somatotrophin extracted from the pituitary glands of human corpses.

Excessive use of somatotrophin could be detrimental, since it can produce physical deformities when taken in adulthood. Large doses produce unnatural enlargement of bones such as jaws, hands and feet, a condition known as *acromegaly*. Nevertheless, Professor Arnold Beckett admits that the drug has created a loophole in Olympic dope control and is currently researching detection methods to enable bans to be enforced[12]. Dr. Robert Voy, chief medical officer of the US Olympic Committee, is also worried about the use of growth hormones. Voy believes that athletes unable to afford human growth hormone are using cut-price extracts supposedly from rhesus monkeys. It may be difficult to establish what these black-market compounds contain, but there may be serious side effects from their use. Fortunately, current developments in genetic engineering have enabled scientists to produce *synthetic* growth hormone. Children with stunted growth should be the first priority for this technical innovation, but there are certain to be athletes who will attempt to get a share in their quest for gold.

Over the last 20 years athletes have developed elaborate and sophisticated techniques to take drugs and avoid detection. The first was to smuggle in a sample of urine given by someone not using drugs. Its disadvantage was that the sample was usually cold, thus arousing suspicion, and it could also produce a few surprises. One male athlete was rumoured to have handed in a urine sample for testing but was caught out when the test revealed the person was pregnant! To overcome this problem the samples must now be collected in containers provided after the event, but again the athletes were one step ahead. They kept a bag of urine belonging to another person, strapped under the arm and kept warm by their own body heat. A tube from the bag ran along the arm inside a jacket, and when the time came to give a sample, operation of a valve emptied the 'safe' urine into the container. It was relatively easy for the athletes to give the impression of behaving normally and the technique became very popular among racing cyclists. Eventually, several cyclists were caught and disqualified, including the Belgian national champion Michel Pollentier and Antoine Guttierez in the 1978 Tour de France. Athletes now have to give urine samples under 'close supervision', and the procedural guidelines for testing have become very complex (see Appendix B).

On the other hand, many athletes have had great difficulty producing samples after their events. Daniel Bautista, the 1976 Olympic gold medallist in the 20,000m walk, was so dehydrated, he had to drink *ten* cans of soft drinks to produce urine for a dope test. Chris Finnegan, the middleweight boxing champion in Mexico, had the same problem. He drank several glasses of water and four pints of beer without the desired effect. The officials eventually received a sample several hours later, which turned out to be negative.

Athletes still try to beat the system by ingesting alkaline solutions such as sodium bicarbonate to alter the pH of the urine. On the other hand, a study by Dr. Bertol and colleagues at the University of Florence revealed how the urinary elimination of doping agents such as amphetamine-like substances, could be modified by the simultaneous ingestion of *acidic* molecules[13]. However, there are important interactions between drugs that may counteract any potential benefits. Another approach has been to use diuretic drugs to increase urine flow and 'flush out' the offending drug before the dope test. Due to the sensitivity of the current testing procedures, most of these tricks can now be caught. Urine samples can be double-checked, by independent laboratories if necessary, and the urine pH or concentration can be altered to overcome any masking strategies.

Since the development of new detection methods, athletes have resorted to other means of artificially improving performance. One technique is known as red blood cell infusion or 'blood-doping'. This came to public attention in 1976, when one of the great athletes of modern times, Lasse Viren of Finland, was asked whether he had been blood-doped. Viren, who was the 5000m and 10,000m gold medallist at both the 1972 and the 1976 Olympic Games, made the celebrated reply that he 'drank only reindeer milk' and later firmly denied the charges. However, rumours about blood-doping have continued, particularly in Finland. In 1981 Mikko Ala Leppilampi, who was fifth in the 1971 European Games and tenth at the 1972 Olympics in the 3000m steeplechase, admitted that he had been blood-doped prior to the 1972 Games[14].

Blood-doping involves the removal of a few hundred millilitres of blood, which is stored for several weeks. The loss of blood stimulates the bone marrow to form more red cells, and the athlete's blood returns to normal in about 3 weeks. The stored red cells are then reinfused a couple of days before the event. In order to function efficiently, muscles must have a constant supply of nutrients and oxygen and the main limiting factor is the ability of the blood to transport oxygen from the lungs to muscle tissue. (Oxygen is carried in the bloodstream by binding to an iron-based pigment in red blood cells called haemoglobin.) Following reinfusion, the extra red cells, and therefore the extra haemoglobin, boosts the oxygen-carrying capacity of the blood, and thus the quantity of oxygen available to the muscles. An infusion of 500ml of blood theoretically adds about 100ml of oxygen to the oxygen-carrying capacity of the bloodstream. A large proportion of the reinfused blood is water, and much of this is removed from circulation, but a large infusion of blood increases the viscosity of the blood, i.e. it is thicker, resulting in decreased cardiac output and blood flow velocity. This slowing of the circulation could reduce peripheral oxygen supply. Therefore, while the blood is 'packed' with extra red blood cells and oxygen, it is taking longer to reach muscle tissue.

While the principles of blood-doping have been known since the early sixties, the first serious research studies that looked at the effects on endurance or performance were conducted in

Sweden, during the late sixties and early seventies by Professor Bjorn Ekblom and his colleagues at the Institute of Physiology of Performance in Stockholm. They initially reported significant and rapid increases in maximum oxygen uptake following blood infusion[8]. They went on to claim that blood-doping increased maximum oxygen uptake by 9 per cent and a *23 per cent* increase in performance[15]. Although some other groups have reported beneficial effects, other researchers have pointed out several problems in the methods commonly used. For example, the Swiss scientists did not use control groups, both subjects and experimenters knew what to expect, and since test-trials took place after blood reinfusion, there may have been a training effect. Other studies reported no improvement in a maximum endurance treadmill run after red cell infusion[16]. Typically, these studies found similar improvements in those 'control' subjects receiving the same volume of a saline solution as the 'experimental' subjects receiving blood infusions. This was despite the fact that the control group would have had lower haemoglobin levels than the experimental group. The improvements observed were probably due to learning or training effects, or the psychological effect of both groups believing they had received a blood infusion, and therefore 'should' perform better. Referring to the lack of evidence to support blood-doping as a reliable means of improving performance, Professor Schonholzer, a member of the FIFA Medical Committee, commented: 'It is quite remarkable how liberally, even negligently, Scandinavian and German scientists have applied these methods and even hastily acclaimed them'.

More recent evidence suggests that it is the amount of blood reinfused which is the critical factor. If only a pint (about 500ml) is withdrawn and reinfused, there is no significant effect on performance. However, if two pints are withdrawn and reinfused several weeks later, some benefits may be obtained. In one well-designed, double-blind study, the times for average runners over a 5-mile (8 km) course were improved by *50 seconds* after blood-doping[17]. It is not likely that such improvements would be found in top athletes. Again, however, it must

117

be emphasised that an improvement of less than a second can make all the difference at this level of competition.

The conclusion that is now emerging is that blood-doping can potentially improve sporting performance, even in well-trained athletes, particularly if adequate precautions are taken to conserve the vitality of the red cells. Despite the criticisms, Professor Ekblom and his colleagues have continued their research, and some of their well-trained athletes have shown 'dramatic' improvements after blood reinfusion[18]. In 1982, Professor Ekblom stated:

> It is with some regret that I conclude that our basic exercise physiology experiments on manipulation of hae-moglobin concentration have some consequences for sport. It is undoubtedly clear, and confirmed by other groups, that by increasing haemoglobin concentration, maximal aerobic power will increase. Central circulation during maximal exercise is mainly unaffected by the rein-fusion. The working muscle can evidently utilise the increased 'offered oxygen' and thus performance is increased.

This conclusion was strongly supported in January 1985 when it was revealed that several members of the American cycling team had been blood-doped prior to the Los Angeles Olympics, at which they won a total of *nine* medals. There had been a period of silence following the Games until Mark Whitehead and a colleague from the American team revealed that half of the team had received an infusion of their own or a relative's blood. The transfusions were reported to have been conducted in a hotel room near the Los Angeles velodrome. Whether the treatment actually improved performance or simply boosted morale cannot be determined. While the director of USOC, Don Miller, condemned the action, an IOC spokesman said that it was unlikely that the cyclists would have to return their medals. However, Jim Hendry, spokesman for the British Cycling Federation, claimed that British cyclists knew that the

Americans had been doped at the time. Indeed one of the British cyclists was told: 'You've got no chance against me to-day, I've had an extra two pints from the milkman'. Hendry urged that blood-doping should be banned[19].

The *New York Times* later accused several other cyclists of being blood-doped. These included Steve Hegg and Leonard Nitz, medallists in the 4000m individual pursuit; Pat Mc-Donough, a member of the silver medal-winning pursuit team; Rebecca Twigg, the women's road-race silver medallist and Brent Emery. All refused to comment on the allegations, but Danny Van Haute, another American cyclist, admitted that he had been blood-doped prior to the Olympic trials.

Blood-doping obviously requires the aid and skills of medical staff, and while it appears straightforward to drain off blood, freeze and store it, and then reinfuse the blood, there are many problems. In all blood transfusion procedures there are inevitable risks including infection and reaction to the anticoagulants used. A certain amount of the frozen blood cells may deteriorate and rupture. This damage to the membrane could provide a clue to detecting athletes who had been blood-doped. Needle-marks on an athlete's arm would only show that they had given or received blood at some time, possibly under conventional circumstances, but if a blood sample was taken and damaged cells were visible under the microscope, this would provide stronger evidence of blood-doping. The amount of cell damage is dependent on the type of freezing technique used. It is likely that the procedure will be perfected in the future and this will make detection even more difficult.

Since adequate tests are not yet available, blood doping is not on the IOC doping list, but the practice has been condemned by the IOC Medical Commission as being against the ethics of sport and possibly dangerous for the athlete's health. There are also substances such as Pentoxyfillin available, that expand the blood vessels and produce an optimum, uniform perfusion of the muscles. While these substances are not prohibited, their use in conjunction with blood-doping would be relatively easy to detect. In March 1985, Prince Alexandre de Merode, chairman of the IOC Medical Commission, announced that the IOC was undertaking investigations into ways of detecting blood-doping.

The prevalence of blood-doping among athletes is not known, but an interesting point was raised by Dr. Daniel Hanley, a member of the IOC Medical Commission[20]. High haemoglobin levels are not necessarily associated with high endurance sports. Oarsmen and runners have often been found to have relatively low haemoglobin levels. In contrast, rifle and pistol shooters, who are sedentary athletes, have haemoglobin levels that are often higher than normal. However, it is quite common for athletes from many nations to go to training camps 'in the mountains' prior to important competitions, and this can affect blood cell concentration. A great deal of research has investigated the effects of exercising at high altitude, and its effects on subsequent performance at sea level.

With increasing altitude the air becomes thinner and the partial pressure of oxygen decreases. The thinner air gives less resistance to people and objects, so many sprinting, jumping and throwing records were broken at the 1968 Olympics in Mexico City, 2300m above sea level. At the Mexico Games, track races were faster than sea level records up to the 800m, in which the world record was equalled, but the longer-distance races were progressively slower. This was almost certainly due to the heat and reduced oxygen availability. At the 1970 World Cup in Mexico, many soccer players from lower-altitude countries became quickly exhausted, despite a period of acclimatisation. Athletes do acclimatise to high altitudes at a rate varying from days to weeks, depending on the altitude. There are several physiological changes to facilitate oxygen transport and utilisation, including increased formation of haemoglobin and red blood cells, but acclimatisation does not fully compensate for the stress of altitude. The maximum volume of oxygen uptake initially decreased about 2 per cent for every 300m above 1500m[21]. This is paralleled by a drop in endurance-related activities. While there are increased red blood cells in circulation, the increased viscosity reduces cardiac output. Even after training at altitude for a number of weeks, performance remains impaired.

One of the most widely accepted myths regarding altitude training is that on returning to sea level, an improvement in performance is guaranteed. Careful and repeated studies have shown no advantage of altitude training on subsequent performance[22]. The athlete's physiology and performance simply returns to normal. Some runners report feeling 'heavy-legged' for some time after their descent. Another widely held belief is that the inhalation of oxygen-rich breathing mixtures prior to, or after vigorous exercise improves performance, but this is not the case. Breathing 100 per cent oxygen *during* performance extends endurance by increasing oxygen uptake and reducing blood lactic acid build-up, but this is obviously impractical for competitive sport.

During exercise, heat has to be transported from deep tissues to the periphery by the blood, but the blood must also deliver oxygen to the muscles. In the intense heat the body can become dehydrated due to excess sweating. Dehydration can reduce the capability of the circulatory and temperature-regulating systems to meet the metabolic and thermal stress of exercise. Marathon runners frequently experience fluid losses in excess of 5 litres during competition, this loss represents 6 to 10 per cent of their body weight, and the fluid has to be replaced to maintain plasma volume so that circulation and sweating can progress at optimum levels. While it would seem reasonable to do this gradually, many athletes feel that ingesting water during a competition hinders performance. In international marathon races prior to the 1976 Montreal Olympics, drinking fluids was prohibited during the first 10km of the race. While fluid replacement is primary during prolonged exercise in the heat, there is no evidence that any drink is preferable to plain water. The more expensive, sugar-containing drinks delay gastric emptying of fluids, which delays the absorption into circulation[23].

There have also been a number of 'nutritional' supplements widely used by athletes with the aim of improving performance. While these are not regarded as doping agents under the present legislation, it is important to dispel many of the myths surrounding their use. Contrary to popular belief, no supplementary salt is needed by sportsmen. There is no evidence that electrolyte intake (e.g. sodium, potassium) during exercise improves performance or reduces physiological strain such as muscle cramps[24]. Under normal circumstances, our dietary intake of salt far exceeds that which is lost through sweating. We already overconsume salt, and additional salt tablets may be dangerous by exacerbating dehydration.

There is some evidence linking overconsumption of salt with the development of high blood pressure. Dr. Norman Kaplan, from the University of Texas in Dallas, argued that there is danger from extra sodium without extra water, due to extreme hypertonicity and kidney failure. He suggested that even those athletes who had to exercise heavily in Los Angeles in August did not need extra sodium[25]. Most of the excess salt consumed in the average Western diet comes from 'junk' food. In those countries where salt intake is low, there is a lower incidence of hypertension and heart disease. A higher incidence of cardio-vascular disorders has been reported in fishing communities in northern Japan, where dietary salt intake is very high, though other factors may be equally important.

On the other hand, some researchers have argued for salt supplementation under *extreme* conditions, such as profuse sweating indoors with ill-ventilated clothing, or intensive exercise in very intense heat. In fact, salt tablets would not only produce nausea or vomiting under these conditions, but would make dehydration worse. However, there are commercial preparations such as 'Slow Sodium' in which the salt is embedded in a wax core that allows a slow release of salt into the intestines, without the sudden gastric contractions which cause nausea[26]. There have been some claims of benefits with these preparations, but it should be emphasised that for most types of sport, we already consume enough salt. Excessive water and electrolyte losses impair heat tolerance and exercise performance, and can lead to severe problems in the form of heat exhaustion, cramps or heat strokes. Since many minerals, including potassium, are lost, athletes use mineral supplements to aid performance. There is no evidence that excess mineral intake benefits performance or enhances recovery after exercise. There are generally adequate amounts of minerals in a well-balanced diet.

Athletic folklore is particularly rich in *vitamin* mythology. It is well known that vitamin supplements will reverse the symptoms of vitamin-deficient states. There is no evidence that taking vitamins will improve any aspect of sporting performance in healthy athletes. Athletes do not have greater vitamin needs than those required by sedentary people. Vitamins are necessary for the maintenance of health, but they do not provide energy and are already generally present in sufficient amounts in our diet. Vitamins regulate metabolism, facilitate energy release and are important in the process of bone and tissue synthesis. However, excess amounts of fat-soluble vitamins (e.g. A, D, E, K) accumulate in the tissues and eventually can be toxic. For example, excess vitamin A can be toxic to the nervous system. Polar bear liver contains very large amounts of vitamin A, perhaps as a result of their fish consumption; the Eskimos discard the liver because it is toxic even in moderate amounts. Also, large doses of vitamin D can damage the kidneys.

Unfortunately, vitamin supplementation is a multimillion pound industry and the advertising is highly effective. While it is unusual for people to take vitamins to the point of toxicity, they are over consumed. Excesses of the water-soluble vitamins (e.g. the 'B' group and vitamin C) are excreted in the urine and it has been suggested that Americans may have the most expensive urine in the world! The belief that 'if a little is good, more must be better' simply does not apply to vitamins, contrary to what is often accepted by coaches, athletes and fitness enthusiasts. It is not supported by controlled scientific studies or by the majority of nutritionists. Studies have revealed that vitamin C supplements had negligible effects on endurance performance compared to treatment with a placebo[27]. Vitamin E has a totally *unwarranted* reputation for increasing athletic and sexual perfor-

123

mance. It has never even been firmly established that a deficiency state for vitamin E exists. While there may be some benefits due to placebo effects, the use of vitamins to improve sporting performance can be summarised by one doctor's comments:

> The sale of vitamins is probably the biggest rip-off in our society today. Their only effect would appear to be a highly enriched sewage around athletic training or competition sites.

While mineral or vitamin supplements are not regarded as doping agents, they do represent substances, that athletes are using to gain a 'competitive edge' over their opponents. They are already present in the body in varying quantities, and are needed for good health. Athletes use other nutritional aids or procedures such as carbohydrate loading or protein supplements, which again is 'legal'.

According to the shot-putter Mike Winch, many of the drug-takers are now *years* ahead of the testing methods[28]. Furthermore, Winch claims that the ability to win medals is dominated to some extent by the quality of the medical back-up. The anti-doping legislation will obviously have to be modified to account for the current changes in doping strategies. The IOC's list of banned substances incorporating the classical stimulants, the narcotic analgesics and the anabolic steroids now cover only a fraction of the substances used. In addition to the problem of blood-doping, future legislation will also have to cover the use of various types of growth hormones, corticosteroids, ACTH, diuretics and 'herbal' products.

8
THE FUTURE

Unless something is done soon, international sport will be a competition between circus freaks manipulated by international chemists.

Peter Lawson, secretary of the UK Central Council for Physical Recreation, 1984.

In a survey conducted by Dr. Gabe Mirkin, over a hundred top American athletes were asked if they were given the option of taking a drug which would make them an Olympic champion but which could kill them within a year, would they take it? Almost *55 per cent* of the sample said they would take the drug[1]. This startling finding not only indicates the value certain individuals place on winning a top sporting event, but perhaps re-emphasises current attitudes towards the use of drugs in sport. For some athletes, winning is all-important, even if it involves risking their health. It also suggests that despite the risk of detection, many athletes would still be prepared to take illegal substances. According to Dr. Albert Dirix of the IOC Medical Commission, there have been at least 30 deaths prior to 1970 directly due to the use of drugs by athletes. The figure is certainly conservative. Worldwide, it is more likely that thousands of athletes have either suffered ill-health or died as a result of using doping agents. It is impossible to assess how many athletes' lives have been ruined as a consequence of doping.

In January 1985, Paul Dickenson, the chairman of the Inter-

125

national Athletics Club, estimated that *60 per cent* of British international athletes are taking some form of drug to enhance performance. While the figure was disputed by Nigel Cooper, secretary of the British Amateur Athletic Board, a worrying problem is that the widespread use of drugs has taken on its own momentum. Doping procedures have changed dramatically since the use of 'strengthening cordials' at the turn of the century, through to the use of stimulants and steroids. Already there are alternative long-term strategies to manipulate physiology such as blood-doping or growth hormone. The artificial manipulation of tendons and muscles to make them more efficient is rapidly becoming a scientific possibility. Techniques are currently being developed to prevent muscle wastage in paraplegics using computer-controlled electrical stimulation of muscles. There may well be spin-offs for the athlete in terms of improving muscle efficiency. There are also rumours of manipulating certain types of muscle fibres by selective patterns of nerve stimulation or 'neural doping'[2].

Will international sport ultimately be contested between 'artificial' athletes aided by scientists from different countries? Will there be sperm banks and ova donated by gold medallists to produce 'preprogrammed' athletes whose growth and development will be geared towards sporting achievement? This conjures up a rather far-fetched image of sport in the future. While this sounds unlikely, the accusations of 'cradle-snatching' by Eastern European sports bodies, whereby potential champions are selected at an increasingly earlier age, begin to read like something from Aldous Huxley's *Brave New World*. It is a chilling thought that we are getting to a point where international sport is concerned only with biologically prepared and pharmacologically manipulated individuals performing to bolster the prestige of particular governments or ideologies.

The underlying reasons may be partially attributed to the fact that we live in a drug-oriented society. Drugs are used to soothe pain, relieve anxiety, help us to sleep, keep us awake, lose or gain weight. For many problems, people rely on drugs rather than seeking alternative coping strategies. It is not surprising

126

that athletes should adopt similar attitudes. In many sports, improved performance is expected to follow from intensive training, sophisticated coaching and monitoring of dietary intake. This requires a great deal of dedication, motivation and hard work. The attraction of taking a substance believed to 'short-cut' all this effort may be very appealing to the less dedicated athlete, and to those wishing to gain an 'edge' over their opponents.

The general availability of drugs can influence what is the 'in' drug for athletes. During the sixties, the availability of stimulants soared during the so-called 'purple heart' era. In Britain, drugs such as amphetamines are controlled drugs such that their supply, possession and import are criminal offences under the 1971 Misuse of Drugs Act. Anabolic steroids fall into a second category, the prescription-only medicines. Their manufacture, import and supply are regulated by the 1968 Medicines Act and require a licence. However, section 13 of this Act permits individuals to import prescription-only medicines for their own use. Furthermore, a substance can be sold as a 'chemical' provided details of dosages or effects are not given. Athletes using drugs-by-post services are acting within the law, providing their purchases are not passed on to third parties. Tightening the legislation further may not solve the problem, since this can create the necessary conditions for a 'black market' trade. David Webster, the Scottish national weightlifting coach and a campaigner against the use of drugs in sport, discussed the availability of steroids and commented: 'If people want them, they can get them quite easily'. Anabolic steroids are certainly widely available at gyms and fitness clubs in Britain.

In several countries it is possible to buy anabolic steroids 'over the counter'. In America, the situation varies from state to state. The USOC group investigating doping describe a publication entitled the *Underground Steroid Handbook for Men and Women*. The 20-page pamphlet, whose unidentified authors apparently lived on the West coast of America, discusses *28* anabolic agents and possible sources[3].

To understand fully the ethical problem of doping, there is a need to re-examine the function of 'sport'. Sport is generally regarded as a recreational pastime or 'diversion' from work, and is an important component in many cultures; but the precise role of sport for any individual is more complex. Sport can be used as means of attaining a state of health and fitness, to meet people, as a means of self-expression or to relieve stress. For many amateur athletes, a 'personal best' is a satisfactory goal. In addition to the pursuit of excellence, especially for the professional or Olympic athlete, the motivations may also be financial or political.

The Ancient Olympic Games were sporting contests, closely allied to a form of religious worship, and initially involving an elite upper class, at which winning athletes could achieve even higher status and favour. When Baron Pierre de Coubertin revived the modern Olympic Games at Athens in 1896, he drew on the English public-school notion of physical competition practised according to unwritten rules of 'fair play'. He believed in amateurism in its purest form, and placed the emphasis on competing rather than winning. The motto that de Coubertin adopted and promoted was written in enormous letters over Wembley stadium for the 1948 Olympic Games. 'The most important thing in the Olympic Games is not winning but taking part. The essential thing in life is not conquering, but fighting well'[4]. But the Olympic movement also has the motto 'Citius, Altius, Fortius' (Faster, Higher, Stronger), apparently demanding elitism and victory. This has placed increasing pressure on the individual to succeed at any cost.

The use of drugs in sport cannot be examined in isolation from the general problems which have afflicted sport. International sport has become increasingly *professional and political*. Both the public and the media in several countries are prepared to acclaim the successful athlete, but they are often equally likely to mock or insult a poor performance. This pressure questions the notion of top international contests being referred to as 'sport' in the true sense of the word. Mike Bull, the British pole vaulter, commented: 'There are so many pressures now on international athletes that even in Britain the good loser is no

longer accepted as a good sportsman'[5]. The American high
jumper, John Thomas, who was expected to win the gold medal
at the 1960 Olympics in Rome, also found that when he came
third, both sports writers and fans turned against him. He said:

> They only like winners. They don't give credit to a man for
> trying. I was called a quitter, a man with no heart. Ameri-
> can spectators are frustrated athletes. In the champion,
> they see what they would like to be. In the loser, they see
> what they actually are, and they treat him with scorn.

Athletes may feel forced to take drugs in order to keep up
with opponents who they believe are taking similar drugs[6]. The
athlete may not only want to compete on a similar par in terms
of drug use, but may even try to outstrip his opponent in the
belief that 'more is better'. There may be an element of bravado
where athletes try to unnerve opponents by hinting at excessive
drug use. The rumours, claims and counter-claims may quickly
spread to such an extent that many athletes take very large doses
of drugs. While the abuse of drugs is widespread, their use is
usually shrouded in secrecy. Athletes are seldom prepared to
discuss the issue publicly, and the silence usually extends to the
coaches, trainers and doctors who are administering the drugs.
Yet when doping reaches the limelight as a result of a disqualification or a death, there are frequent claims that drug use among
athletes in that sport was 'common knowledge'. If this is the
case, it is important to question why sporting journalists have
not spoken out on the subject, or why officials from that sport
have not introduced regular dope-testing.

In international sport, there are relentless pressures on athletes from coaches, trainers, sponsors and even governments.
Certain countries with few social, economic or scientific
achievements, or countries who want to demonstrate the superi-
ority of their socio-economic system, *use* sport to increase their
prestige. Sporting success can be manipulated by governments
to reflect the personal characteristics of their peoples or the
quality of their social system. Thus the promotion of sport has

become a major political concern, and if success is believed to be possible through the use of drugs, then drugs are used. It is possible that in some countries, athletes, coaches or doctors, not believing in the ethics or benefits of doping procedures, may be *forced* to use them.

In December 1978 the 20-year-old East German sprinter, Renate Neufield, revealed that she had had regularly been forced by East German coaches to take drugs. She experienced a range of unpleasant side effects including abnormal hair growth and menstrual disturbances. When she refused to take the drugs, Neufield claimed she was interrogated, and alleged that there were threats of reprisals aimed at her and her family. Neufield defected to the West in 1977 after the 'psychological pressures' became too intense. She brought samples of the drugs to West Germany, where they were identified by Professor Donike of the West German Sports Federation as anabolic steroids[7].

There have been other defectors with similar stories to tell. Thus the Western media portray an image of Eastern bloc countries in which athletes perform under conditions of reprisal, and doped physically with drugs or psychologically through hypnosis. While it is true that drugs and hypnosis have been used in Eastern European countries, the same is also true for the West. Whatever the political ideology, the stakes in international competition are high. Victory brings increased status for the individual, his family, results in financial and career rewards and boosts the image of the country. Defeat can result in personal humiliation, a loss of a career and does nothing for the image of the athlete's country.

The West also portrays the Eastern bloc's 'preparation' of athletes as plucking potential champions from schools at an early age and awarding them various opportunities to enable them to train[8]. However, is the situation so different in the West? Athletes may be helped through sponsorship, advertising, sporting scholarships at prominent universities, or simply given time off work to train. That countries then go on to flout doping regulations cannot be disputed; it is simply that in some

130

countries it is conducted more covertly. Indeed, it has been argued that drug use in Eastern Europe is 'safer' in that it is more controlled than in countries where athletes rely on black market sources.

In 1981 Paul Nevala, Finland's javelin champion in the 1964 Olympics, accused the country's sports administrators of covertly permitting drug abuse among athletes[9]. Nevala claimed that excessive doses were commonly used and commented: 'I used them myself during two years of my career, and they finished me'. Citing the mysterious deaths of three Finnish girls at training camps, Nevala maintained that sports managers knew full well that these potentially lethal bodybuilding substances were in wide circulation. Linda Haglund, the top Swedish sprinter, claimed that she had been given drugs without her knowledge by her Finnish coach. Haglund was banned after a positive dope test at the Swedish championships. In June 1985 Dr. Marku Alen of Jyvaskyla University claimed that Finnish competitors who won 13 Olympic medals in Los Angeles had used banned substances. Dr. Alen also said that 71 Finnish contestants used illegal stimulants while training for the Games, but refused to reveal the names of the offenders.

In Britain, the secretary of the Central Council for Physical Recreation, Peter Lawson claimed that 12- and 13-year-old children were taking drugs to improve performance[10]. There was an outcry from Members of Parliament who called for an inquiry. In August 1981 Dr. David Cowan, assistant director of the Chelsea College Drug Testing Centre, highlighted the case of a boy aged 13 who had been given a stimulant, without his knowledge, by his coach. The boy thought the treatment was for pain relief; the names of the people involved were not revealed[11].

As well as the risks and side effects, the use of drugs by children may be damaging in shaping their attitudes. Most youngsters set the top athletes of the day on a pedestal, and wish to emulate their feats. If they are led to believe that drug use in sport is normal, they will readily accept it. The first step should be to educate young athletes concerning the effects of

131

drugs, the dangers and the legislation. If this proves to be inadequate, then drug testing may have to be introduced into athletic competition at a much earlier stage. Indeed in October 1984 ten swimmers aged between 12 and 19 were called on for dope-testing during the Hewlett-Packard English Schools swimming championships at Morden, Surrey. They were drawn at random, one each from 10 of the 11 finals, and parents and coaches were permitted to be present. According to Fred Uglow, secretary of the English Schools Association, 'There had been no pressure on us to do the testing. With a drug problem among youth throughout the country, we hope to show the world that we are not troubled by it'[12].

There is much superstition and rumour concerning 'wonder-drugs' among athletes, and the 'experimentation' for effects may be based on nothing more than speculation or hearsay. Other competitors may feel that they have done everything possible both physically and mentally to prepare themselves for the event, but still feel that they must do more. The use of drugs could be regarded as adding a new dimension to their prep-aration. While anti-doping legislation often seems to implicitly accept that doping can have a positive effect on standards, the preceding chapters have illustrated how the effects of drugs on performance can be highly variable, depending on the indi-vidual, the side effects, or the dose used.

In 1980 Sir Arthur Gold, president of the European Athletics Association, commented: 'Sport is about health and honesty, taking drugs is unhealthy and dishonest'[13]. In addition, many sportsmen and women have spoken out against the use of drugs in sport. In particular, the 1984 gold medallist, Ed Moses of the USA, one of the greatest hurdlers of modern times, has cam-paigned for all sports to be free of doping practices. Howard Payne summed up the feelings of many competitors when he commented:

In terms of athletic morals it is better that we remain poor in the field events rather than we achieve artificial results through doping. To my mind, the person who uses these anabolic steroids in athletics is as despicable as the cheat who knowingly uses a light discus in competition.

Nationally, some countries have already used legislative powers to ban doping in sport: France and Belgium since the sixties, Italy and Turkey in 1971 and Greece in 1976. In other countries, national sport confederations have imposed binding regulations on their members, notably the Swiss Sports Association since 1967, the Deutsche Sportbund and the Norwegian Confederation of Sport in 1977, the Danish Sports Federation in 1978, the Swedish Sports Federation and the Finnish Sports Federation in 1982. Since the IOC introduced dope-testing in 1968, various international federations, starting with the Union Cycliste Internationale, have adopted anti-doping regulations, generally based on those of the IOC. For their own part the IOC and IAAF have a jointly agreed system of accreditation of laboratories to guarantee the testing procedures match the standards required, and hopefully to ensure they are politically trustworthy. The accredited laboratories are mainly concentrated in Europe, the exceptions being Montreal and Los Angeles.

The control of doping rests primarily with the national governing bodies, and sports federations may eventually be pressured into spending even more money on anti-doping projects. In September 1984 the Swedish Sports Confederation announced that it was to spend around 230,000 pounds on a campaign against drug abuse in sport. This followed the disqualification of two Swedish athletes at the 1984 Olympic Games; Thomas Johannson, the Greco-Roman wrestling silver medallist, and Goran Pettersson, who was sixth in the heavyweight weightlifting contest. The money will enable drug tests to be held more frequently, to improve specialist hospital facilities, and improve education about drugs for young athletes[14]. The announcement coincided with an admission from Frank Andersson, a Swedish former world wrestling champion, who claimed he had used drugs before winning the European title in 1978 and later before the 1980 Olympic Games.

The Council of Europe has been aware of the dangers of doping in sport since the early sixties. In the European 'Sport For All' Charter defined by the 1st Conference of European Ministers responsible for sport in Brussels, 1975, the member states agreed to take measures 'to safeguard sport and sportsmen from practices that are debasing and abusive, including the unfair use of drugs'. The problem was also discussed at the 2nd Conference of Sports Ministers in London, 1978. The outcome was the Council of Europe's 'Anti-Doping Charter for Sport' which was accepted by Sports Ministers at their meeting in Malta during May 1984.

The anti-doping charter stresses that the elimination of drug misuse in sport will require common action by public authorities, each acting within the sphere of its own responsibilities and the Council recommends the governments of member States:

- to implement effective anti-doping regulations,
- to create and operate doping control laboratories,
- to encourage and promote suitable research in these drug testing centres,
- to devise and implement educational campaigns against drug misuse,
- and to assist with the financing of doping controls.

The Council of Europe also recommends its member States to encourage their national sports organisations:

- to adopt the IOC and IAAF anti-doping regulations, procedures and lists of banned substances,
- to make full use of existing doping control facilities,
- to introduce compulsory drug testing for all their national standard members,
- to impose substantial penalties on those members proven guilty of drug misuse,
- to take similar action against others assisting or enticing them, and finally to review unnecessarily high qualifying standards for national and international events.

The charter aims to make a European contribution to a problem which affects sport worldwide. Effective action against doping requires co-operative action, not only between governments and non-governmental organisations, but more important, *internationally*. Unfortunately, this co-operation does not exist at present at several of the levels required.

Many sporting organisations still refuse to accept that drug use could be a potential problem in their sport, and therefore do not see the need for doping regulations or dope testing. According to Mrs. A. Williams, Chief Administrative Assistant of the Amateur Swimming Association, 'as far as we are concerned, there is "no use of drugs" in swimming'[15]. Similarly, Mr. R. L. Clarke, General Secretary of the British Boxing Board of Control, commented,

> we have had no experience of boxers taking any form of dope or drugs, in fact it is a strict regulation of ours that no kind of stimulant must be taken by our boxers before or during a contest[16].

But stimulant use is only one type of doping practice, and one that is now regarded as rather passe. There are several drugs that could obviously be used by boxers either to lose or gain weight, to ensure being in a particular weight category prior to a bout. If these are not tested for, how can the boxing authorities be sure they are not being used? Mr. Clarke added

> Our rules do not call for dope tests although these could be undertaken if it was ever suspected. In European and World Championships that take place in this country, a dope test is mandatory. This has always been carried out and to date there has never been a positive result.

Other sports have started dope-testing relatively recently. Following preliminary tests in 1978, the Badminton Association of England announced it would test for the first time at

135

the 1979 All-England Championships at Wembley, while according to the Squash Racket Association's Chief Executive, Mr. R. I. Morris, the Association

> is actively urging the International Federation to institute a list of proscribed drugs which could enable member countries to conduct random drug tests. I suspect that next season will see the first drug testing in squash[17].

Dick Jeeps, former chairman of the British Sports Council, commented on the 'apathy, ignorance and evasion' of some sporting bodies with respect to drug abuse[18]. While certain sports were taking significant steps to stamp out drug abuse, Mr. Jeeps pointed out that expense was 'no excuse' for the others, since the Sports Council gave 100 per cent subsidies for drug testing. Over the past 5 years the Council has spent 500,000 pounds on the drug testing programme, research and funding of the Drug Control Centre at Chelsea College. At the start of 1984, only *14* of the 60 governing bodies under the Sports Council's umbrella were using the free drug-testing facilities, so in March 1984 they decided to step up the campaign. The Council is now considering withdrawing their grants from governing bodies who refuse to introduce random drug testing[19]. John Wheatley, the Council's Director-General, commented: 'We mean business with these new measures. We don't want to take financial sanctions against any sport, but it is one of the options we shall have to consider'. The number of sporting bodies using, or proposing to use, the facilities currently stands at 25, which still only represents less than half of the total number.

In March 1985 the Sports Council stepped up its anti-drug campaign even more. It was announced that by June 1985, every sport must inform the Council what testing arrangements they are making, and grants would be withdrawn after December 1985 if there had been no adequate response.

In addition to improved co-operation between governments,

sports federations and organisations, there is a need to re-
examine anti-doping legislation, the manner in which the tests
are conducted and the punishments if positive tests are revealed.
Firstly, there are slight discrepancies between the IOC and
IAAF regulations, the use of codeine being the most obvious
example. The time required to modify the list of banned substances needs to be reduced. At present, a period of 3 years is
needed for each international federation requesting either an
addition or a modification to the list. After this time, athletes
may have moved on to other types of drugs. Secondly, and
more importantly, the tests need to be *random*. If athletes are
using stimulants, then they are likely to use them on the day of
the event, and then would be the obvious time to test for them;
but if athletes are using anabolic steroids, testosterone or
growth hormones, their use is over a period of weeks or
months. They could stop taking them several weeks prior to the
event to avoid detection. The only way to test these athletes is at
random during their training periods.

Following the disqualification of two Russian oarsmen at the
1980 Mannheim regatta, the president of the International
Rowing Federation, Thomi Keller, spoke out on the need for
random testing during training periods[20]. In Britain the Amateur Rowing Association conduct 'swoop' dope-tests, but Dr.
Martyn Lucking has emphasised that random testing must be
worldwide in order to be effective. Financed by the Sports
Council, Dr. Lucking has conducted research on behalf of the
International Athletes Club. He claims that random testing
would be a greater deterrent to drug users, and ultimately
would be cheaper, because fewer tests would be required.
Furthermore the testing of *top* athletes only at *top* competitions
only serves to reinforce the myths that these are the athletes
most likely to have used drugs.

, The solution may be to have international dope-testing
squads who, under the guidance of the IOC or international
federations, travel from country to country and test athletes
randomly during their training throughout the year. This is
already the case in the Scandinavian countries where indepen-

dent officers set up by governments can ask for a sample from an athlete at any time in competition or training.

In February 1985 the British Amateur Athletic Board announced that random drug testing was to be introduced for all British athletes and only those competitors who agreed to have their names included on a register to be tested would be eligible for international competition. The secretary, Nigel Cooper, claimed the voluntary register and testing programme would show the world that doping was not a problem in British sport. Sir Arthur Gold had proposed a similar register for all Olympic competitors 2 years earlier. The suggestion was greeted with silence by the governing bodies of most sports. Are other countries likely to follow Britain's example?

Given the present political climate and the level of mistrust and suspicion between East and West, the chances are very slim. Whenever particular athletes perform brilliantly, or appear to have unusually muscular physiques, suspicions of doping arise. This was certainly the case at the Moscow Olympics in 1980, with respect to the East German women's swimming team[21]. The East Germans were first, second and third in both the 100m freestyle and 100m butterfly events. In the freestyle event all three were at least 2 seconds clear of the rest of the field, a remarkable margin at this level of competition. The East German women dominated the swimming events. They were particularly well-built and some observers suggested that anabolic steroids or testosterone had been used. The suspicions were strengthened by the fact that the remarkable domination was only evident in the female short-distance events, where muscle mass and power are crucial. However, none of the swimmers concerned failed the dope tests.

Some observers have suggested that countries not agreeing to random dope-testing should not be allowed to participate in major competitions. Others disagree and suggest that this would create major and minor leagues of competing nations. The situation could become very complex, particularly if athletes from 'tested' countries spent most of their training periods in countries where testing was not permitted.

The importance of random testing was highlighted when six athletes were withdrawn after being positively dope-tested *prior* to the 1985 European Indoor Championships in Athens. The results, which were announced on the night before the events began, stunned both the organisers and the Greek government who had sponsored the event. The six athletes, five men and a woman, all professed their innocence. Less than a week later Dr. Antonis Koutselinis confirmed that *14* Greek athletes were found to have taken banned substances.

The Sports Medicine Division of the United States Olympic Committee (USOC) administered drug tests prior to the Olympic Games at their Olympic Trials. All those who were selected were tested according to IOC guidelines, and any positives were disqualified. According to Bob Beeten, manager of the Clinical Services for USOC, 'the only deviation is that a sport can request informal testing some months prior to the Trials, these results have no penalty if they are positive'[22]. It is difficult to see the purpose of this procedure. An athlete should not be using doping substances at any time, so why should the testing be penalty-free at this time, precisely the period when an athlete could potentially be bodybuilding with the help of testosterone or anabolic steroids? Indeed, rather than deterring doping, this 'service' could inform the anxious athlete whether traces of steroids were detectable well before the Trials, and without any fear of being penalised. Following the Games in Los Angeles, the USOC organised a study committee, directed by Dr. Kenneth Clarke, to examine the results of their drug testing programme and to make further recommendations for future Games.

In January 1985 it was revealed that *86* American athletes had failed doping tests before the Los Angeles Games. Over 2000 athletes were tested; and 33 were found to have used stimulants and 53 had used steroids. Ten of the athletes who failed were screened during the Olympic trials and two had already won places in the American team. Don Miller of USOC regarded the programme as a 'success' because no American athlete failed doping tests at the Games. While it is true that no American athlete failed tests for steroids or stimulants, American competitors *were* guilty of using beta-blockers and being blood-doped!

There are limitations on the effectiveness of current doping controls, but a statement in 1978 by Sir Arthur Gold is particularly ominous:

> I have been reliably informed that in the recent Commonwealth Games in Edmonton, management officials of two large teams not only connived with but actively assisted some of their athletes to evade doping controls. Learning that there would be random testing on arrival in the village, they kept their athletes out of the village as long as possible, and in the case of one team, treated possible positives with diuretics and systematically flushed them with vast quantities of fluids[23].

An incident reported by the Paris journalist, Eric Lahmy further illustrates the problem[24]. The incident apparently occurred at the end of a stage in an unnamed major cycling race. When asked to be tested, all the cyclists admitted that they had used the drugs, and therefore all should be disqualified. Faced with the dilemma, the organisers, doctors, officials and journalists gave in and the incident was hushed up. While cyclists have been prime offenders in the past, the situation seems to be improving.

The British Cycling Federation impose a ban of 6 months for a first doping offence, 2 years for a second offence and a life ban for a third offence. Some observers have argued that the penalty for the first offence is too lenient but it is possible that the drug was used as a consequence of ignorance or stupidity. It is easy to retest first offenders to determine whether they are habitual users, and if so, they pay the price by receiving a longer sentence. This seems to be a sensible system, and importantly, the British Cycling Federation largely carry out *random* testing, rather than testing just at major events. If riders fail to turn up for a test, they are treated exactly as though they had produced a positive sample. Bryan Wotton, the secretary of the Federation said:

> In recent years, we have been fortunate in mostly obtaining negative samples and whilst we are not complacent, we are certainly confident that there is very little misuse of drugs within the sport of cycling in the UK[25].

According to Mr. Wotton, there are only three British riders currently under suspension for failing to attend a medical control. The British Cycling Federation have conducted dope-testing regularly since 1965, long before the Sports Council subsidies, and despite some unfortunate press publicity now appear to have the situation under control.

In contrast to the British regulations, the Union Cycliste Internationale require that amateur riders be suspended for a period of 1 month for a first offence, 6 months for a second offence and confiscation of their licence for a third. Professional cyclists are fined and given a suspended sentence of 1 month for a first offence, a second offence results in a fine and a 3-month suspension, and confiscation of their licence for a third offence. The British regulations do not make a distinction between amateur and professional riders.

While federations are obviously concerned about the welfare and success of their athletes, they are also concerned about the image and prestige of their sport and the consequences for possible sponsorship or financing from advertising. If anti-doping regulations are to be successful, they must have the support of the various federations to enforce *consistent* penalties for *all* the guilty parties, doctors, coaches or trainers. The function of dope control is essentially to constitute a deterrent rather than a punishment.

The anti-doping charter suggests that sports organisations should be encouraged to agree on similar and substantial penalties for sportsmen or women caught using doping substances and for any person providing, administering or facilitating the use of doping substances. At the 1981 Olympic Congress the

141

athletes called for a life ban on athletes, coaches, or doctors using or administering prohibited drugs. There are cases where athletes have accidentally taken a medication containing prohibited substances, such as Ron Angus or Rick DeMont. Nevertheless, there have been others fully aware of the risks and penalties involved, who were still prepared to take illegal substances. There are also those cases where athletes claim that they were doped by their coaches without their knowledge. This raises the possibility of athletes using the coach as a 'fall guy'.

There is still controversy over what constitutes a 'substantial' penalty for athletes guilty of doping. The English Olympic Wrestling Association registration form states 'Any member of the association taking drugs to improve performance automatically suspends him or herself for life'[26]. If athletes appeal, life bans are seldom enforced. Athletes are usually reinstated between 1 and 2 years later by their national federations. The reinstatement can be even quicker, as illustrated by the return of the disqualified Balkan athletes prior to the 1980 Olympic Games. When an American world record holder in the discus was banned after a positive test, not only did the American Federation refuse to enforce the ban, they made him their Athlete of the Year. Similarly, in a French pre-Olympic skiing competition, two Austrian women were found guilty of doping, but the ban was not enforced by the Austrian authorities, and one of then went on to win a medal at Sarajevo[27]. This interference by a sporting federation clearly undermines the IOC anti-doping campaign.

When several weightlifters from various countries were disqualified at the Montreal Olympics in 1976, the IOC threatened to exclude weightlifting from future Games, if the International Weightlifting Federation did not conduct its own tests. The tests were conducted, but only at the end of major weightlifting competitions. The offenders were not deterred and weightlifters have continued to be disqualified for drug use, as shown at both the 1983 Pan-American Games and the 1984 Olympic Games.

In September 1981 the National Collegiate Athletic Association (NCAA) conducted a confidential survey of athletes at ten large universities located in the upper-midwest of the United States. The findings, published in August 1982, examined the use and attitudes to drugs among 1000 male student athletes in football, basketball, track and swimming teams. Almost *95 per cent* of the athletes claimed they had never used drugs to improve performance[28]. It is impossible to generalise from this pilot study to all student–athletes, but the NCAA is currently funding a major research project to gather data from a larger sample of both male and female athletes. While the NCAA survey suggests that a relatively small number of American student athletes take drugs to improve performance, the pressures to succeed are only beginning at this stage. If a place in an Olympic team was at stake, it is certain that many more would be tempted. Indeed, this NCAA finding should be contrasted with a statement from an American coach who commented 'It's my honest belief that 75 per cent of the women in the American team are not taking drugs'. The implication of the statement is that a *quarter* of American women athletes *are* taking drugs.

The point was reinforced by Daley Thompson, the Olympic decathlon champion, during a television interview in March 1985. Thompson estimated that while one-third of Britain's athletes have taken drugs, the figure was as high as 80 per cent in the United States. He added 'It is a lot more serious than people think, the problem needs to be tackled'.

In 1980 a survey was conducted by Dr. Peter Radford, director of the Department of Physical Education and Recreation at the University of Glasgow[29]. He was interested in how athletes viewed the role of 'sports scientists', and his survey questioned both club athletes and British track and field athletes at the Moscow Olympics. The athletes were well aware of the benefits of sports science, and believed that it will become even more important over the next 10 years, but they generally felt that there are fewer knowledgeable sports scientists in Britain than in other leading sporting nations.

Dr. Radford found the 'undisguised amorality' among some

143

athletes' views on sport particularly worrying. Athletes made comments such as 'I am only interested in sports scientists if they can give me an advantage over other athletes', or 'Athletes will use whatever methods are available, the sports scientist should check to see it is done safely'. The survey illustrated how many athletes felt that the presence of sports scientists tends to reduce the pleasure of sport and make it more of a 'business'.

The sports scientists are placed in a very difficult situation, since there appears to be a growing tension between investigators seeking to expand knowledge, and those seeking 'practical' information that can be 'used' to better results for political ends[30]. In addition athletes do not always accept the findings of the scientists. When presented with data suggesting a particular drug does not improve sporting performance, some athletes will continue to use that drug. Even when presented with case histories illustrating the dangers of using the drug, athletes may still accept the risk. Other athletes may have difficulty obtaining information demonstrating insignificant effects of doping procedures on performance, since many scientific journals tend not to publish 'negative' findings.

Prince Alexandre de Merode, president of the IOC Medical Commission, is realistic about the future of doping in sport. He admits

Cheating will go on to the end of the world, but our job must be as much to expose the health dangers, of depression, of glandular and cardiovascular damage, as to ban people.

In modern international sport, Prince de Merode insists that there is already too much competition for the human body to endure. He suggests that the number of hours spent in athletic training should be limited by regulation, just as in other forms of working employment[31]. The difficulties of enforcing such types of regulation would be immense.

In December 1983 Neil Macfarlane, the UK Under-Secretary of State for the Environment, stated 'Doping is perhaps the most pernicious and intractable problem in sport today'[32]. Indeed, it seems unlikely that doping will ever be *totally* eliminated from international sport. Modern international sporting events, including the Olympic Games, induce a show of excess patriotic fervour, chauvinism and jingoism and there are many with a vested interest in maintaining this system. Since the public seldom divorce the individual performance from the national origin of the competitor, it is difficult to foresee the depoliticisation of future international sport. Perhaps the time is rapidly approaching to step back and re-assess what 'sport' is all about. The misuse of drugs is not only a health hazard, but is contrary to the ethics of sport and the ideals of sportsmanship and fair play. To ensure that athletes are not tempted to use drugs, they have to be convinced that dishonour is not in defeat. Otherwise, sport is in danger of becoming trials of misapplied science rather than trials of human talent and ability.

9
OVERVIEW

Throughout this book we have tried to be objective in describing the extent and nature of drug abuse in sports. Nevertheless, readers will be aware that, although this is an accurate account, we have tended to emphasise the undesirable consequences of drug abuse, rather than the purported benefits. However, not everyone would agree with our bias. This short chapter outlines some of our reasons for taking this stance and explains why we believe drug abuse is bad for the future of sport.

There are many people, including athletes, coaches and doctors, who do advocate drug use in sports and they have their own arguments to support their position. Typically, such people claim that the extent of the 'problem' is not very great and/or the health risks are of no significance. The truth is that, as this book has shown, the problem is enormous; drug abuse is ubiquitous in sports. Indeed we have probably reached the point where the remaining 'clean' sports are very much in the minority. Regarding the dangers, there are certainly fewer deaths due to drug abuse in sport than to, for example, hang-gliding or motor racing, where a moment's lapse of attention may be fatal. Even with indoor sports the risks are sometimes considerable: there have been over 60 deaths on squash courts during the last 6 years. The supporters of drug use would say this puts drug-related health risks into perspective. Actually, such comparisons are absolutely meaningless; these statistics are completely independent of each other. It is equally ridiculous to compare the number of drug-related deaths with, for example, those caused by malaria. Certainly some sports are dangerous but the risk is an inherent aspect of the sport. Drug-related risks are both additional and unnecessary. Surely the most important point is that competitors *have* died as a result of taking drugs in order to improve their sporting performance; the actual number is not the issue. Perhaps those people who see this purely in terms of numbers should ask themselves how many deaths are necessary to make this problem an important one. The preceding chapters have demonstrated that the problem of drug abuse *is* widespread, and while there is no evidence of an 'epidemic' of drug-related deaths in sports, the health risks from using drugs in such enormous doses should be a concern to us all.

Many people would raise the objection that by regulating against drug use we are denying sportsmen and women their fundamental right to choose their training methods. For example, some would argue that if research showed that athletes' performances could be improved by drugs they should be free to use them. If there were any risks or side effects the athletes could be warned. Such people feel that this is no different to making use of the best available diet or technique. Hence a drug might be regarded simply as another tool at the athlete's disposal. If we regard drugs as a legitimate means of augmenting performance then dope-testing denies athletes the freedom of choice. These arguments are not acceptable for many reasons. While it is true that many athletes are fanatical about their health and pay meticulous attention to their diet and training, they are still prepared to take potentially harmful substances in the hope of gaining that vital edge. The number of illnesses and deaths testify to this fact. Furthermore, because such drugs are used illicitly athletes have difficulty obtaining accurate information and many are *unaware* of the risks associated with drug abuse. More worrying is the attitude among many top athletes that 'winning isn't everything, it is the *only* thing!' which means

that, even when the risks are obvious, drug abuse could continue unabated.

It could be argued that many of us already abuse dangerous
substances, for example alcohol and tobacco, in our daily lives;
if these are acceptable then why not allow drug use in sports?
We believe the two situations are simply not comparable.
People who drink alcohol are usually aware of the risk to our
brains and livers, but we are able and prepared to take that risk.
While there may be social pressures to drink or smoke, the
choice ultimately belongs to the individual. By abstaining from
these 'recreational' drugs it is unlikely that we will suffer in any
way; in fact the opposite is probably true. The athlete's decision
about performance enhancing drugs is very different. In reality
athletes have no choice. It does not matter whether the drug
'works', if one competitor *suspects* another of having taken a
new drug, or a higher dose of an existing one, then he or she
will feel pressured to follow. The realisation or suspicion that
your competitors have access to drugs when you do not could
be so demoralising that you are beaten before you start. In an
environment where milliseconds or centimetres determine the
difference between winner and loser, any advantage, or
imagined advantage, is a powerful factor. Thus while many
athletes feel it is they who are making the choice the decision
has already been taken for them as soon as one competitor turns
to drugs.

In other situations the athlete's decision may be influenced in
a more sinister way. Young naive athletes may be easy victims
for unscrupulous coaches while the financial and political pressures exerted by sponsors and governments may cajole the
sportsman into drug abuse. Unless they are truly exceptional
athletes their choice about drugs may simply be either to take
them or leave the competition. The fact that some athletes
actually do get to the top without resorting to drugs is reassur-
ing, but will that be the case in the future?

The athlete who decides to take steroids, or the person who
chooses to drink alcohol every day, may be risking their *own*
health but what of those people who take drugs that may

endanger others? For example, those who opt to smoke in confined spaces may be harming the health of those around them who do not smoke. More dramatically, American footballers may not like to face a team whose defenders were highly aggressive 'speed freaks'. So, in the contact sports, taking drugs to enhance rage and aggression must be regarded as a dangerous and socially irresponsible act.

The dedication shown by all sportsmen and women is incredible. They may spend years training for an event which may last only a few seconds so they cannot afford to take any chances. If this means that athletes are dependent on drugs for their performance then the outcome of sporting events will ultimately be determined by chemists with the athletes serving merely as pawns. This is clearly not what sport, at any level, is about.

It has also been argued that if pharmacologists were able to develop drugs that were 'safe and effective' then athletes should be free to make use of them. While drugs may be 'safe and effective' within their therapeutic dose range, there are many examples of problems which arise as the dose is dramatically increased. If we examine the past use of drugs in sport there is abundant evidence that athletes do not keep to recommended dose levels. If 'safe and effective' drugs were introduced we believe athletes would use higher and higher doses in order to gain an advantage over their competitors. Most substances are toxic if taken in large enough amounts and athletes simply do not know when to stop. Also, the expression 'safe and effective' is dependent on the current state of our knowledge. Several 'safe' drugs have been introduced which have proved to be absolute disasters after some years of their use.

Thus over and above the inequality that exists between individuals, teams or countries, doping should be regarded as an unfair and often dangerous means of attempting to improve performance. We have already indicated the difficulty of determining which drugs are 'fair' when it comes to sports. Drugs are needed to reduce pain and aid recovery from illness or injury; athletes are prone to the same disorders as the rest of us and need the same array of drugs. They are also entitled to use

149

or abuse 'recreational' drugs if they so desire. Clearly, we are not objecting to the rational use of drugs for therapeutic reasons; our concern is that drugs are not used irresponsibly, without appropriate supervision, with the specific intention of augmenting sporting performance. We believe it is unethical and undermines the spirit of sport; it may also eventually lead to the physical damage of athletes or their fellow competitors. This distinction between the use and abuse of drugs is clear in theory but very complex in practice. For example, some athletes will continue to compete despite very painful injuries, while others may take analgesics to alleviate their pain. How can officials decide when an injury is painful enough to warrant the use of analgesics? If it is, what type of analgesic? There are similar problems in deciding when an anti-anxiety agent should be regarded as a doping agent. How can one distinguish between the marksman who has a stiff drink the night before competition to help him sleep, and his competitor who has the same drink immediately before the event to steady his hand?

There are obviously many 'grey areas' with respect to the specific use of drugs in sport but there are many more with respect to other types of physiological manipulations. Is the starving of female gymnasts to retain their prepubertal 'elfin' appearances so different from giving boxers drugs to cause weight loss? The end result is surely the same. We feel that both are unnecessary strategies and each may bring its own problems. For example, the high incidence of anorexia nervosa among gymnasts may be partially attributed to the intensity of competition and preoccupation with body weight and image. What is different *is* that while it would not be possible to legislate against dietary manipulations without enormous difficulty, it is feasible to test for drugs. This is the key factor in anti-doping legislation. There is no point banning alcohol or caffeine as these are used by almost everyone. Similarly all men have different levels of testosterone. All that officials can do is decide on what is the 'normal' range and test for levels outside that range. Other, more arbitrary, decisions have been made; for example, all narcotics, anabolic steroids and stimulants are banned in sport yet some anti-asthmatic agents, which share certain properties with the stimulants, are permitted.

In taking a stance against drug abuse in sports we are not attacking sports science. Sports science has a great deal to offer the serious athlete. Exercise programmes designed to develop specific groups of muscles can be an important component of training; slow-motion video analysis or computer simulations may be important in improving technique; biofeedback and relaxation training can be an essential aspect of psychological preparation for competition. The list is long and wide-ranging. The use of drugs in sports, i.e. sports pharmacology, is only one branch of sports science. It is a fascinating area and is as honest a topic for research and as laudable an expression of human achievement as, for example, atomic physics. However, in the wrong hands the former has given us the chemical athlete and the latter the threat of nuclear war and global destruction. Neither of these outcomes can be blamed exclusively on scientists. We, as a society, must shoulder the responsibility for the way science is managed. Nevertheless, scientists should be acutely aware of the possible consequences and implications of their research, including any possible abuses. We believe that most forms of sport science *are* legitimate (despite the fact that athletes do not have equal access to this technology) but we have singled out sports pharmacology as an area which, unfortunately, has been dramatically abused.

There are two aspects to athletic competition: winning medals and breaking records. If a record is set by one individual who has had some chemical assistance then this is surely no different to an athlete who cheats by using a light javelin, shot or discus. If the drug has had the desired effect then the record may not be broken for many years except by another drug-user. The situation is rather different for events where all competitors are taking the same drugs; the probability is that, while the overall standard of performance will increase, the way the athletes are ranked will not change. We seem to be rapidly approaching this situation; the only way for individuals to gain an advantage is to experiment with higher doses and wider

151

combinations of drugs. Ostensibly the answer to the problem is to ensure that no-one takes drugs; however, it is not as easy as this. Where the stakes are so high there will always be someone who is prepared to risk disqualification. The problem will always be with us for as long as we put so high a value on winning as opposed to competing. Also, although it would help if penalties for drug use were extended to coaches, team physicians and selectors this would not obviate the possibility of a calculated official attempt to flaunt the regulations. Many Western athletes already accuse certain Eastern bloc countries of doing just this. Ultimately we have to rely on the integrity of the individual to act according to his or her own conscience; the future of sport is in serious jeopardy if this chemical war continues. Sport is about *honest* competition. Either we accept this and persuade athletes to forsake their tablets and syringes or we forget about the honesty. With chemicals in the stadium it is a rat race, not a human one.

Appendix A
The Autonomic Nervous System

Our nervous system can be regarded as consisting of the *central* and the *autonomic* nervous system. The central nervous system consists of the brain and spinal cord. The brain receives and sends messages via the spinal cord to the muscles which cause movement, the skeletal or 'voluntary' muscles. In contrast, the autonomic nervous system supplies the *viscera*, such as the heart, lungs, stomach, intestines, blood vessels and various secretory (or endocrine) glands. In brief, the central nervous system controls voluntary actions while the autonomic nervous system controls vegetative processes such as heart rate, blood pressure and digestion. The autonomic nervous system is controlled (via the pituitary gland) by an area at the base of the brain called the *hypothalamus*. Since it receives information from the rest of the central nervous system, the hypothalamus can be regarded as providing the link betwen the activity of the central and the autonomic nervous systems.

The autonomic nervous system can be further subdivided into two parts, the sympathetic and parasympathetic systems, which generally have opposite effects on the organs they supply. The parasympathetic system is 'dominant' during periods of inactivity such as sleep, relaxation or meditation. In this resting state, heart rate and blood pressure are lowered, and we feel calm (see Chapter 6). However, when we are more active or 'threatened' in some way the sympathetic system is activated. We are all aware of the feelings associated with fear or anger. The heart pounds, our breathing becomes rapid, we may experience a sinking feeling in our stomach, and we may start trembling or sweating. This classic 'fight, or flight' response prepares the body to cope with some threat or danger. This 'stress' response may have helped our ancestors to escape from predators.

When the sympathetic system is activated, heart rate is increased and blood vessels are constricted. The overall effect is to increase blood pressure and thus to increase the oxygen supply to the muscles. The increased supply of blood to the skin causes the characteristic red face associated with anger, while the redistribution of blood away from the face characterises fear. Other sympathetically mediated effects include dilation of the pupils, decreased gastric activity and elevated blood sugar levels. Thus the body's energy resources are 'mobilised' and we are prepared to tackle whatever initially caused the response.

When the autonomic system is activated via signals from the hypothalamus and pituitary gland, a substance is released at the nerve endings in the tissues concerned. The pattern is different for the sympathetic and parasympathetic systems in terms of the anatomical systems involved and the transmitting substances used. When the sympathetic system is activated, the hormones, noradrenalin and adrenalin are released from the adrenal glands. These enter the bloodstream and are circulated around the body. When noradrenalin and adrenalin reach tissues such as heart, lungs, or blood vessels, they produce the effects shown in Table A.1. Corticosteroids are also released from the adrenal cortex which increase the supply of glucose to the blood and generally speed up metabolic rate. Although the sympathetic system is activated in times of fear, a not uncommon parasympathetic symptom in extreme emotion is the involuntary emptying of the bladder or bowels.

While the effects of the sympathetic and parasympathetic systems appear to be antagonistic, they actually work in close co-operation. For example, if you are sitting in the sun eating a meal the sympathetic system will promote sweating, while the parasympathetic system will promote digestion. In male sexual

TABLE A.1

	Parasympathetic	Sympathetic
Heart rate	Decreased	Increased
Bronchi	Constricted	Dilated
Saliva flow	Stimulated	Inhibited
Pupils	Constricted	Dilated
Peristalsis	Increased	Decreased
Secretion of digestive juices	Increased	Decreased

behaviour the erection is 'parasympathetically mediated' while ejaculation is a 'sympathetically mediated' response. Thus normal behaviour depends on complex interactions between the two systems. Some of the effects of parasympathetic 'activation' are also shown in Table A.1.

Appendix B
Rule 29 of the Olympic Charter

Medical code

1.1. Doping is forbidden. The IOC shall prepare a list of prohibited drugs.

1.2. All Olympic competitors are liable to medical control and examination carried out in conformity with the rules of the IOC Medical Commission.

1.3. Any Olympic competitor refusing to submit to a medical control or examination or who is found guilty of doping shall be excluded. If the Olympic competitor is a member of a team, the match, competition or event during which the infringement took place shall be forfeited by that team.

After the explanations of the team have been considered and the case discussed with the International Federation (IF) concerned, a team in which one or more members have been found guilty of doping may be excluded from the Olympic Games in which it is participating.

In sports in which a team may no longer compete after a member has been excluded, the remaining members may compete in an individual capacity.

1.4. Female competitors must comply with the prescribed tests for femininity.

1.5. A medal may be withdrawn by order of the Executive Board on a proposal of the IOC Medical Commission.

1.6. A Medical Commission may be set up to implement these Rules. Members of this commission may not act as team doctors.

1.7. The above regulations shall in no way affect further sanctions by the IFs.

PROCEDURAL GUIDELINES

1. *Selection of athletes*

1.1. A reasonable number of doping controls shall be undertaken in all sports.

1.2. The number of athletes to be checked per day in each sport shall be agreed upon by the IOC Medical Commission, the International Federation concerned and the Orgainising Committee, with due consideration to the available laboratory capacity.

1.3. The International Federation concerned shall determine the number of athletes in the various events of its sport to undergo a control, in accordance with the total number agreed upon under section 5.1.2.

1.4. Before the end of the competition, the International Federation concerned shall likewise determine the criteria for selecting the competitors to be checked.

1.5. If doping is suspected, the IOC Medical Commission shall have the right to demand additional athletes be checked.

1.6. An athlete may be tested for drugs on more than one occasion during the Games.

2. *Sample-taking procedure*

2.1. Immediately after the contest or after determination of the final results, the competitor selected for a doping check shall be handed a testing notification by a representative of the Organising Committee who should accompany the competitor to the waiting-room of the doping control station designated on the testing notification. The competitor must report to the doping control station as soon as possible within the hour with his identity card.

The testing notification shall bear the competitor's starting number and the statement that an attendant (team official, coach or doctor) may be present when the competitor is reporting to give a sample; moreover, it shall point out the possible consequences if an athlete should fail to report for the control within the time limit. Part of the notification shall be a detachable stub which shall also bear the competitor's starting number and shall confirm that the competitor has taken note of the representative's request.

2.2. When the representative has entered the time on the main part of the notification and on the detachable stub, the competitor shall sign the notice of confirmation on the stub.

2.3. The representative shall pass the stub to the official in charge of the doping control station concerned.

2.4. Should the competitor fail to report to the doping control station within the time set in section 7.2.1, the fact shall be noted in the records. The records shall be signed by the official in charge of the station and shall be delivered immediately through the chairman of the Doping Control Committee to the chairman of the IOC Medical Commission, or his representative. The IOC Medical Commission shall decide on the further procedures to be followed.

2.5. Upon arrival at the doping control station, the competitor and the accompanying person shall be attended in the waiting room by a member of the doping control team.

2.6. The representative of the Organising Committee shall check the identity of the competitor by means of the identity card and the starting number.

2.7. Whenever possible, only one competitor at a time shall be called into the doping control office to provide a sample.

2.8. In addition to the competitor and the accompanying person, only the following persons may be present in the doping control office:

– the official in charge of the station,
– a medical technician, whose duties include keeping the records,
– a representative of the International Federation concerned,
– a member of the IOC Medical Commission, or a person nominated by it.
– the official in charge of taking samples,
– an interpreter.

2.9. The time and the personal data of the competitor shall be noted in the records.

2.10. The competitor shall select an unused urine collector in a sealed bag.

2.11. The competitor shall urinate (at least 75 ml) into this collector under the supervision of the person responsible for taking the sample.

2.12. If the competitor refuses to give a sample of urine, the possible consequences shall be pointed out to the athlete. If the competitor still refuses, this fact shall be noted in the records. These shall be signed by the official in charge of the station, the medical technician, the competitor, the representative of the international federation concerned, and the accompanying person (if any), and shall be sent immediately through the president of the Doping Control Committee to the chairman of the IOC Medical Commission.

2.13. If the competitor is unable to gie an ample urine quantity after a fair period of time, this fact shall be noted in the records. The procedure decided by the Medical Commission of the IOC shall then be followed.

2.14. Immediately following the taking of the sample, the competitor shall select another sealed bag which contains two bottles. The competitor shall pour approximately an equal amount of urine into each bottle and shall close them securely.

2.15. The official in charge of the station, after verifying that the two bottles are well closed, shall code them with a control number selected by the competitor and shall seal them.

2.16. The official in charge of the station shall give the

competitor and the accompanying person an opportunity to make sure that the bottles are correctly sealed.

2.17. The code number shall be noted in the records by the official in charge of the station. The medical technician shall give the competitor and the accompanying person an opportunity to ascertain that the number noted in the records agrees with that recorded on the two bottles.

2.18. The competitor shall certify by signing the records that there have been no irregularities in the entire sample taking procedure. The records shall also be signed by the official in charge of the station and the accompanying person (if any), and shall be placed in separate envelopes and sealed.

2.19. The envelope containing the original copy of the records shall be sent throgh the chairman of the Doping Control Committee, to the chairman of the IOC Medical Commission. For security reasons the duplicate copy shall be kept sealed, in a safe, unless released by the Chairman of the IOC Medical Commission, or his representatives.

2.20. The medical technician shall place each of the bottles in separate containers which shall then be sealed immediately.

2.21. All the sealed containers, each holding a sealed bottle, shall be placed in a special box which itself shall be sealed in the presence of witnesses who shall sign the records annexed to the box before it is transported to the laboratory.

2.22. This sealed box shall be given to the courier upon signature of a receipt which will indicate the number of samples in the box, the site from which they come and the departure time of the courier.

2.23. The courier shall take the sealed box to the laboratory immediately.

2.24. At the laboratory, a person appointed by the head of the laboratory shall ackowledge receipt of the sealed boxes. This person shall take note of the time of arrival.

APPENDIX B

3. *Sample analysis*

3.1. The analysis of a sample shall be completed as soon as possible after its arrival at the laboratory.

3.2. The analysis of a sample shall be carried out according to well-established methods which have been approved by the IOC Medical Commission.

3.3. In addition to the head of the laboratory and the laboratory staff, only the following persons shall be admitted to the laboratory during analysis:

– Members of the IOC Medical Commission.
– Persons with special authorisation from the IOC Medical Commission.
– The chairman of the Doping Control Committee.

3.4. Should the analysis prove positive, the head of the laboratory shall immediately inform the chairman of the IOC Medical Commission or his representative.

3.5. The chief of the delegation to which the competitor belongs, or his representative, shall be immediately informed in writing by the chairman of the IOC Medical Commission or his representative, that the analysis of the first sample has proved positive and that the second sample will be analysed at the time determined by the IOC Medical Commission, which will be as prompt as possible.

3.6. The analysis of the duplicate sample shall be carried out in the same laboratory but by different persons. The analysis shall be supervised by a member of the IOC Medical Commission. The delegation in question shall be allowed to send a maximum of three representatives to the laboratory. The member of the IOC Medical Commission shall inform the Chairman of the Commission of the result of this analysis.

3.7. Should the result be positive, the Chairman of the IOC Medical Commission shall then, without delay, call a meeting of the IOC Medical Commission to which a representative from the international federation concerned and the chairman of

161

the Doping Control Committee will be invited. If he/she so desires the athlete may be heard at this meeting.

3.8. The Chairman of the IOC Medical Commission shall pass the recommendation of the IOC Medical Commission to the President of the IOC who will be responsible for taking the necessary action. The head of the delegation to which the competitor belongs will also be informed.

3.9. The result of this control analysis shall be final.

4. *Femininity control*

4.1. The femininity control of all the women's sporting events of the XIVth Olympic Winter Games shall be carried out in accordance with the decisions and instructions of the Medical Commission of the IOC. The result of this examination will not be made public out of deference to the human rights of the individual.

4.2. Competitors who have been registered as females must report to the femininity control head office. Those competitors who fail to report cannot take part in the Games.

4.3. The test will be set up at the Olympic Village under the supervision of a member of the IOC Medical Commission.

4.4. In the name of the Medical Commission, the femininity control group will notify each chief of the mission or his representative of the day and time of the test for his team.

4.5. The delegation representative who has been notified will have the responsibility of seeing that their women competitors present themselves with their identity cards at the examination room on the day and time appointed, accompanied by an interpreter (if necessary).

4.6. Female competitors who have a valid certificate of femininity, which has been issued by the IOC Medical Commission, will be exempted from another examination upon presenting that certificate to the femininity head office.

4.7. The identification of the competitor appearing for the control will be made by the identity card and will include the competitor's photograph, weight, size and accreditation number. In some cases, the individual's passport could also be requested.

4.8. As a screening test, the determination of X and Y chromatins will be conducted on a smear of buccal mucous membrane.

4.9. If the test is inconclusive, the competitor must undergo further tests as determined by the IOC Medical Commission.

4.10. The results of the examination will be reported to the chaiman of the Medical Commission or his appointed representative only.

4.11. Should the results of these tests require it, the chairman will call a meeting of the Medical Commission at which a physician from the team and a representative of the International Federation concerned may be present, following which a physical examination can be prescribed and performed by a physician gynaecologist member of or accepted by Medical Commission.

4.12. The Medical Commission will issue a femininity certificate to those competitors whose test results are conclusive.

Approved on February 14, 1983 in Sarajevo by the IOC Medical Commission and on June 21, 1983 in Lausanne by the IOC.

Appendix C
Detection of Anabolic Steroids

Stage 1: Radioimmunoassay

This is a technique now widely used in the biological sciences for detecting the presence of particular chemical entities. Basically what happens is this. Anabolic steroids are chemically bound to a protein and this combination is injected into an animal, usually a rabbit, which reacts to the protein/steroid combination as it would to any foreign substance: it produces antibodies to protect itself. These antibodies attach themselves quite specifically to a particular protein/steroid combination. By using radioactive labelling the presence of anabolic steroid in a urine sample can be detected. There is always a small amount of 'cross-reactivity' in this method (i.e. the specificity for a particular steroid cannot be guaranteed) but this is not a problem since the next stage identifies the steroid(s) present.

Stage 2: Gas Chromatography/Mass Spectrometry

Although this is technically very complicated it is based on quite simple principles. The urine sample is first put through a 'clean-up' procedure to remove some of the unwanted chemicals that would otherwise interfere with the assay. This is then concentrated and a portion is injected into a device called a gas chromatograph. This separates the remaining components of the mixture and passes them into a mass spectrometer through a special interface. Here the components of the sample are broken down and passed through a magnetic field which 'focusses' the breakdown products according to their mass and ionic charge. A 'fingerprint' of each component can be built up in this way, allowing specific steroids to be identified and measured.

References and Notes

In writing this book, we have drawn on a wide range of articles from medical and scientific journals and textbooks, British newspapers, (particularly *The Times*, *The Sunday Times* and the *Guardian*), popular magazines, radio and television programmes and press releases. In addition we have contacted people, clubs, sporting organisations and governing bodies directly. We have tried to acknowledge these sources of information whenever possible.

Chapter 1: Introduction

1. Finley, M. I. and Plecket, H. W. (1976) *The Olympic Games: the first hundred years*, Chatto and Windus, London.
2. Hanley, D. F. (1983) *Clinical Sports Medicine*, **2**, 13–17.
3. The International Amateur Athletics Federation (IAAF) simply define doping as 'the use or distribution to an athlete of certain substances which could have the effect of improving artificially the athlete's physical and/or mental condition and so augmenting his athletic performance'. IAAF Doping Control Regulations and Guidelines for Procedures, Rule 144, 1982.
4. The historical examples were taken from several books and articles, e.g.
Brant, M. (1980) *The Games*. Proteus, London.
Cuddon J. A. (1980) *The Macmillan Dictionary of Sport and Games*. Macmillan, London
Emery, D. (ed.) (1984) *Who's Who in the 1984 Olympics*. Pelham Books, London.

Goldman, B. *et al.* (1984) *Death in the Locker Room.* Century Books, 1984.

Woodland, L. (1980) *Dope: the use of drugs in sport.* David and Charles, Newton Abbot.

Shephard, R. J. (1978) *The Fit Athlete.* Oxford University Press, Oxford.

Thomason, H. (1982) 'Drugs in sport'. In: Davis, B. and Thomas, G. (eds) *Science and Sporting Performance: management or manipulation?* Clarendon Press, Oxford.

Matthews, P. (1982) *The Guinness Book of Athletics: facts and feats.* Guinness Superlatives, London.

Holt, R. (1981) *Sport and Society in Modern France.* MacMillan, London.

Harris, N. *et al.* (1982) *The Sports Health Handbook.* World's Work.

Wallechinsky, D. (1984) *The Complete Book of the Olympics.* Penguin, Harmondsworth.

5. Personal communication, November 7th, November 27th 1984.
6. Sports Council Press Release, 22nd May 1978.
7. The weightlifters involved were Zbigniew Kaczmarek of Poland, Dragomir Ciorosian of Romania, Blagoi Blagoev and Valentin Hristov of Bulgaria, Petr Pavalsek of Czechoslovakia, Mark Cameron and Philip Grippaldi of USA.
8. Reports in *The Times*, March 13th, May 1st, June 5th and November 1980; *The Sunday Times*, August 3rd 1980.
9. Report in *The Sunday Times*, July 6th 1980.

CHAPTER 2: STIMULANTS

1. *IOC Medical Guide*, 1984.
2. Reports in the *Guardian*, June 1984. In April 1985, Livingstone Bramble, the WBA lightweight champion was fined $15,000 for having ephedrine in his bloodstream during his successful title defence against Ray 'Boom-Boom' Mancini. David Wolf, Mancini's manager said he would petition the WBA for Bramble's disqualification, however, he is unlikely to be successful.
3. Karpovich, P. V. and Sinning, W. E. (1971). *Physiology of Muscular Activity.* W. B. Saunders, Philadelphia.

4. For example: Bhaghat, B. and Wheeler, N. (1973). *Neuropharmacology*, **12,** 711–713.

   Gerald, M. C. (1978) *Neuropharmacology*, **17,** 703–704.

5. Smith, G. M. and Beecher, H. K. (1959) *Journal of the American Medical Association*, **170,** 542–557.

   Smith, G. M. and Beecher, H. K. (1960) *Journal of the American Medical Association*, **172,** 1502–1514.

6. For example: Karpovich, P. V. (1959) *Journal of the American Medical Association*, **170,** 558.

   Golding, L. A. and Barnard, R. J. (1963) *Journal of Sports Medicine and Physical Fitness*, **3,** 221.

7. Chandler, J. and Blair, S. (1980) *Medical Science and Sports*, **12,** 65.

8. For example: Foltz, E. E. *et al.* (1943) *Journal of Laboratory and Clinical Medicine*, **28,** 601.

   Haldi, J. and Wynn, W. (1959) *Research Quarterly*, **17,** 96.

   Hurst, P. N., Radlow, R. and Bagley, S. K. (1968) *Ergonomics*, **11,** 47–52.

   Wyndham, C. H. *et al.* (1971) *South African Medical Journal*, **45,** 247.

9. Laties, V. G. and Weiss, B. (1981) *Federation Proceedings*, **40,** 2689–2692.

10. In mice, this drug causes increased aggression and better motor co-ordination, but a 40 per cent *reduction* in swimming endurance (see Estler, C. J. and Gabrys, M. K. (1979) *Psychopharmacology*, **63,** 281–284.)

11. One drug scandal involved the championship-winning Everton team of the early sixties; however, such stories are difficult to substantiate. We wrote to a number of clubs in the First and Second Divisions of the English League. Those clubs that replied (Arsenal, Coventry, Manchester United, Tottenham Hotspur and Wolverhampton Wanderers) all stated that they were unaware of any use of drugs by soccer players.

12. Personal communication from FA and EUFA, April 5th 1984. Report in the *Daily Telegraph*, March 29th 1979.

13. Marshall, E. (1979) *Science*, **203,** 626–628.

14. Mandell, A. J. (1976) *The Nightmare Season*. Random House, New York.

15. Mandell, A. J., Stewart, K. D. and Russo, P. V. (1981) *Federation Proceedings*, **40,** 2693–2698.

Also see Mandell, A. J. (1978) *Journal of Psychedelic Drugs*, **10**, 379–383.

Physician and Sportsmedicine, September 1973.

16. As a result of his appeal to the State Superior Court regarding the Medical Quality Assurance Board's decision on June 2nd 1980, the Superior Court of California ordered that the decision in the matter of the accusation against Mandell, dated October 31st 1977, be set aside. The probation was lifted and he was in effect exonerated on all counts. Mandell commented 'I've stayed as far as possible from the NFL since those days. The issues are still not resolved but the problems haven't been going away. . . .' (Personal communication, December 28th 1984).

17. Lawton, J. (1984) *The All-American War Game*. Blackwell, Oxford.

    Goldman, B. *et al.* (1984) *Death in the Locker Room*. Century Books.

    In April 1985 several *basketball* players from Tulane, USA were involved in a scandal involving cocaine and bribery.

18. Bouton, J. (1970) *Ball Four*. Bell.

    In May 1985 a Federal grand jury in Pittsburgh revealed its findings concerning drug taking by baseball players. Nearly two dozen players, including the pitcher Vida Blue, have been publicly involved in drug-related incidents since 1980. However, the Major League Baseball Players' Association has resisted the idea of drug testing on the grounds that it would 'dehumanise' players.

19. Cooper, D. L. (1972) *Journal of the American Medical Association*, **221**, 1007–1011.

20. Reports in *The Times*, November 1984.

    Report in the *Guardian*, October 15th 1984.

21. *IOC Medical Guide*, 1984.

22. Costill, D. L. *et al.* (1978 and 1979) *Medical Science and Sports*, **10**, 155–158; and **11**, 6–11.

23. For example: Perkins, J. *et al.* (1975) *Medical Science and Sports*, **7**, 221–224.

    Berglund, B. *et al.* (1982) *International Journal of Sports Medicine*, **4**, 234–236.

    Essig, D. *et al.* (1980) *International Journal of Sports Medicine*, **1**, 86–90.

    Lopes, J. *et al.* (1983) *Journal of Applied Physiology*, **54**, 1303–1305.

    Schade, E. *et al.* (1979) *Federation Proceedings*, **38**, 944.

169

Also see: Delbecke, F. T. and Debackere, M. (1984) *International Journal of Sports Medicine,* **5,** 179–182.

24. *IOC Medical Guide,* 1984.
25. Report in *The Times,* October 18th 1982.
26. Dr. Billy Patton, Nottingham University Oral History Project (personal communication, 1984).

CHAPTER 3: ANABOLIC STEROIDS

1. An anabolic steroid is a steroid which promotes tissue growth. There are many types of steroid all of which share a common basic ring structure, as shown in Figure 3.2.
2. The force generated by a muscle is related mainly to muscle cross-sectional diameter but other factors influence the relationship. For example, we are often not able to activate all the fibres in a muscle – someone who can achieve this may show greater strength than another with bigger muscles but who cannot. Also, women tend to produce more force than men relative to their muscle size. Intense training for a woman may result in large increases in strength but relatively little increase in muscle diameter.
3. The results that Dr. Solberg (1983) reported *(British Journal of Sports Medicine,* **16,** 169–171) show an increased improvement rate in lifting records during the 1960s and early 1970s. His claim that this 'came to an end around 1976' is not supported by his evidence, since the rate of improvement appears not to change from 1973 to 1982. Consequently, his idea that the sale of steroids is related to the rate at which records are set cannot be substantiated. This is not to deny that there is such a relationship; it is likely that Solberg's data on steroid sales are misleading in that unofficial (black market) sales must have increased after the 1976 ban on their use.
4. Ryan, A. J. (1981) *Federation Proceedings,* **40,** 2682–2688.
5. Freed, D. *et al.* (1975) *British Medical Journal,* **2,** 471–473.
6. Alen, M., Hakkinen, K. and Komi, P. V. (1984) *Acta Physiologica Scandinavica,* **122,** 535–544.
7. Capes, G. (1981) *Big Shot. An Autobiography.* Stanley Paul.
8. According to Professor David Lamb (personal communication, 1984), 'there are as many different stacking regimens as there are

athletes. As one might expect the outstanding chemical athletes tend to have their favourite 'stacks' mimicked by their followers'.

9. Wright, J. E. (1980) *Exercise and Sport Science Research*, **8**, 149–202.

10. Lamb, D. R. (1984) *American Journal of Sports Medicine*, **12**, 31–38.
    In this report Professor Lamb summarised the results of 19 well-controlled clinical studies on anabolic steroids. Twelve of these showed more weight gain in the steroid-treated groups, on average about 2.2kg. The duration of the trials was from 3 to 12 weeks with doses of methandienone up to 100mg/day. Professor Lamb could offer no explanation as to why steroids increase body weight in some studies but not others. Similarly, with weightlifting performance he drew the same conclusions as Drs. Ryan and Wright in that only half the experiments showed improvements as a result of steroid treatment.

11. Haupt, H. A. *et al.* (1984) *American Journal of Sports Medicine*, **12**, 469–84.

12. Kochakian, C. D. and Murlin, J. R. (1935) *Journal of Nutrition*, **10**, 437–459.

13. Professor G. R. Hervey (1982) makes the point that oestrogenic steroids are usually used in commercial meat production (G. R. Hervey, 'What are the effects of anabolic steroids?' In: *Science and Sporting Performance: management or manipulation?*, p. 131, Clarendon Press, Oxford); but one of the more popular veterinary products, trenbolone, is actually androgenic. Athletes are already using trenbolone and claim noticeable strength increases.

14. Analysis of muscle tissue has led some people to the opinion that anabolic steroids 'inflate' the muscles with water and salts (e.g. Hervey, G. R., see note 13 above). Others have performed a different type of biopsy and believe that the steroids build true muscle fibres (e.g. Alen, M. *et al.* (1984) *Acta Physiologica Scandinavica,* **122**, 535-544).

15. Sklarek, H. M. *et al.* (1984) *New England Journal of Medicine*, **311**, 1701.

16. Goldman, B. *et al.* (1984) *Death in the Locker Room*. Century Books.

17. In deciding 'how much is too much' we run into statistical problems. Because officials want to discipline only the guilty athletes they have to ensure that anyone who has *naturally* high levels of testosterone is not penalised. Clearly these naturally high levels will overlap with the lower levels of athletes who have had

171

testosterone injections. In making sure all the 'clean' athletes get through the net it is inevitable that some of the 'dirty' ones will evade detection.

CHAPTER 4: DRUGS AND THE FEMALE ATHLETE

1. Pannick, D. (1983) *Sex Discrimination in Sport*, an Equal Opportunities Commission booklet, UK.
2. Wade, P. (1983) *Winning Women*. Queen Anne Press MacDonald & Co., London and Sydney.
3. The studies of sexuality in adrenalectomised women are open to criticism as the adrenals are only removed in cases of terminal cancer. Such women might be expected not to show much interest in sex anyway so investigations of their libido are questionable. Despite this the evidence from work on monkeys strongly suggests a role for adrenal androgens as mediators of female sexual urges.
4. Diddle, A. W. (1983) *Southern Medical Journal,* **76,** 619–624.
5. Aleb Acheed, L. *et al.* (1982) *Journal de Gynecologie, Obstetrique et Biologie de la Reproduction,* **11,** 697–701.
6. Goldman, B. *et al.* (1984) *Death in the Locker Room.* Century Books.
7. The nuclei of living cells contain genetic material (chromosomes) which determines how that cell will develop. The chromosomes are arranged in pairs – the number of pairs depending on the organism in question. Humans have 23 pairs of chromosomes, one pair of which are sex chromosomes. If the two sex chromosomes are matched then the owner is female (XX), if they are not matched then it is male (XY). At least two X chromosomes are needed for the cells to display Barr bodies (named after their discoverer Murray Barr), so men do not have them.
8. Wallechinsky, D. (1984) *The Complete Book of the Olympics.* Penguin, Harmondsworth.
9. Hughes, R. *The Sunday Times Magazine*, May 20th 1984.

CHAPTER 5: ANTI-ANXIETY DRUGS

1. For example, Burgen, A. S. V. and Mitchell, J. P. (1978) *Gaddums Pharmacology,* Oxford University Press, Oxford.

172

2. Personal communication, April 9th 1984.
3. Report in *The Sunday Times*, March 23rd 1980.
4. Report in *The Times*, September 26th 1983.
5. Reports in *The Times*, October 12th, November 14th and 22nd 1984.
6. Steadward, R. D. and Singh, M. (1975) *Medical Science and Sports*, **7,** 309–311.
7. Report in *The Times*, October 18th 1980.
8. Personal communication, April 11th 1984.
9. For example: Sperryn, P. (1983) *Sport and Medicine.* Butterworths.
Cratty, B. J. (1973) *Psychology in Contemporary Sport.* Prentice Hall, New York.
Rushall, B. S. (1979) *Psyching in Sport.* Pelham, London.
Straub, W. F. (ed.) (1980) *Sport Psychology: an analysis of athlete behavior.* Movement Publications.

CHAPTER 6: PAINKILLERS

1. Melzack, R. (1973) *The Puzzle of Pain.* Penguin, Harmondsworth.
2. For review, see Gardiner, P. F. (1983) *The Physician and Sports Medicine,* **11,** 71–73.
3. *IOC Medical Guide*, 1984.
4. Reports in *The Times*, February 27th and April 12th 1983.
5. Reports in *The Sunday Times*, May 15th and December 4th 1983.
Reports in *The Times*, December 5th and 30th 1983.
6. Woodland, L. (1980) *Dope: the use of drugs in sport.* David and Charles, Newton Abbot.
7. Matthews, P. (1982) *The Guinness Book of Athletics: facts and feats.* Guinness Superlatives, London
8. For example: Feight, C. B. *et al.* (1978) *Lancet,* **ii,** 1145–1146.
Warren, M. P. (1980) *Journal of Clinical Endocrinology,* **51,** 1150–1157.
Carr, D. B. *et al.* (1981) *New England Journal of Medicine,* **305,** 560–563.
Howlett, T. A. *et al.* (1984) *British Medical Journal,* **288,** 1950–1952.
9. McMurray, R., Sheps, D. S. and Guinan, D. M. (1984) *Journal of Applied Physiology,* **56.**

10. Carlson, N. R. (1980) *Physiology of Behavior.* Allyn and Bacon.
11. *Psychology Today,* May 1984.
12. Melzack, R. and Wall, P. (1982) *The Challenge of Pain.* Penguin, Harmondsworth.

CHAPTER 7: CURRENT TRENDS

1. Woodland, L. (1980) *Dope: the use of drugs in sport.* David and Charles, Newton Abbot.
   Shephard, R. J. (1978) *The Fit Athlete.* Oxford University Press, Oxford.
2. Report in *The Times,* November 4th 1983.
3. Fulder, S. (1980) *The Root of Being.* Hutchison, London.
   Report in *The Sunday Times,* July 20th 1980.
4. Fulder, S. (1980) *New Scientist,* **87,** 576–579.
5. Avakian, E. V. and Evonuk, E. (1979) *Planta Medica,* **36,** 43–48.
6. Schneider, S. H. *et al.* (1981) *Metabolism* **30,** 590–595.
7. Lamb, D. R. (1984) *Physiology of Exercise: responses and adaptations.* Macmillan, New York.
   Jones, N. L. *et al.* (1977) *Journal of Applied Physiology,* **43,** 959–964.
   Kinderman, W. *et al.* (1977) *European Journal of Applied Physiology,* **37,** 197–204.
8. *IOC Medical Guide, 1984.*
9. Report in *The Times,* October 18th 1980.
10. Reports in the *Guardian,* September 1984.
11. Reports in *The Times,* November 15th and 24th 1983.
    Also see: Taylor, W. N. (1985) *Hormonal Manipulation: a new era of monstrous athletes.* McFarland.
12. Report in *The Sunday Times,* June 3rd 1984.
13. Bertol, E. *et al.* (1980) *Journal of Sports Medicine,* **20,** 383–386.
14. Matthews, P. (1982) *The Guinness Book of Athletics: facts and feats.* Guinness Superlatives, London.
15. Ekblom, B. *et al.* (1972, 1976) *Journal of Applied Physiology,* **33,** 175; **40,** 379.
16. Williams, M. H. *et al.* (1973, 1978) *Medical Science and Sports,* **5,** 181; **10,** 13.
17. Williams, M. H. *et al.* (1981) *Medical Science and Sports Exercise,* **13,** 169–175.

REFERENCES AND NOTES

18. Ekbolm, B. (1982) In: Davis, B. and Thomas, G. (eds) *Science and Sporting Performance: management or manipulation?* Clarendon Press, Oxford.
Gledhill, N. *et al.* (1978) *Medical Science and Sports*, **10**, 10.
19. Reports in the *Guardian*, January 1985.
20. Hanley, D. L. (1979) In: R. H. Strauss (ed.) *Sports Medicine and Physiology*. W. B. Saunders, Philadelphia.
21. McArdle, W. D., Katch, F. I. and Katch, V. L. (1981) *Exercise Physiology*. Lea and Febiger, Philadelphia.
22. For example: Adams, W. C. *et al.* (1975) *Journal of Applied Physiology*, **39**, 262.
23. Coyle, E. F. *et al.* (1978) *Research Quarterly*, **49**, 119–124.
24. Costill, D. L. *et al.* (1975) *Aviation, Space and Environmental Medicine*, **46**, 795.
25. Kaplan, N. M. (1984) *Journal of the American Medical Association*, **252**, 528.
26. Sperryn, P. N. (1983) *Sport and Medicine*. Butterworths, London.
27. Gey, G.O. *et al.* (1970) *Journal of the American Medical Association*, **211**, 105.
28. Report in *The Times*, November 4th 1983.

CHAPTER 8: THE FUTURE

1. Northern Ireland Institute of Coaching article.
2. Shepard, R. (1982) In: Davis, B. and Thomas, G. (eds) *Science and Sporting Performance: management or manipulation?* Clarendon Press, Oxford.
3. Gunby, P. (1984) *Journal of the American Medical Association*, **252**, 454–460.
4. While the Olympic motto is usually attributed to Baron de Coubertin, it was actually first propounded by a Bishop of Pennsylvania in a different context.
5. Bull, M. (1974) *Athletics Coaching*, **8**, 4.
6. Ryan, A. J. (1984) *Journal of the American Medical Association*, **252**, 517–519.
7. In: Woodland, L. (1980) *Dope: the use of drugs in sport*. David and Charles, Newton Abbot.
8. For excellent accounts of how sport is regarded and conducted in the Soviet Union, see the following books by James Riordan.

175

Riordan, J. (1977) *Sport in Soviet Society*. Cambridge University Press, Cambridge.

Riordan, J. (ed.) (1978) *Sport under Communism*. C. Hurst, London.

Riordan, J. (1980) *Soviet Sport: background to the Olympics*. Blackwell, Oxford.

The latter is particularly useful in dispelling many of the myths that have been created or fuelled by the media in the West concerning sport in the USSR.

With respect to the use of drugs in sport in the Soviet Union, the 'official line' is that the problem exists only in the West. Cases of Soviet athletes being disqualified for doping offences are seldom reported in the media. However, it is likely that doping is a major problem in the Soviet Union, although it is difficult to prove. It is also difficult to determine how available certain drugs such as anabolic steroids are likely to be in the Soviet Union. The fact that Soviet coaches have attempted to buy them while competing in the West suggests that perhaps they are not as available as popularly believed. As in the West, their use is usually shrouded in secrecy.

9. Report in *The Times*, March 22nd 1981.
10. Reports in *The Times*, September 15th and 16th 1978; also see *The Times Educational Supplement*, February 20th 1981.
11. Report in *The Times*, August 6th 1981.
12. Report in *The Observer*, October 28th 1984.
13. Report in *The Times*, October 18th 1980.
14. Report in the *Guardian*, September 1984.
15. Personal communication, November 5th 1984.
16. Personal communication, November 2nd 1984.
17. Personal communication, April 16th 1984.
18. Report in *The Times*, November 4th 1983.
19. Sports Council Press Release, March 27th 1984.
20. Reports in *The Times*, July 19th and October 18th 1980.
21. Report in *The Sunday Times*, July 27th 1980.
22. Personal communication, May 15th 1984.
23. In: Woodland, L. (1980) *Dope: the use of drugs in sport*. David and Charles, Newton Abbot.
24. Lahmy, E. Journalist, *L'Equipe, Paris*.
25. Personal communication, November 27th 1984.
26. Personal communication, November 21st 1984

27. Report in *Woman*, August 1984.
28. Personal communications, April 30th and September 7th 1984.
29. Radford, P. (1982) In: Davies, B. and Thomas, G. (eds). *Science and Sporting Performance: management or manipulation?* Clarendon Press, Oxford.
30. Shepard, R. In: Davies, B. and Thomas, G. (see note 29 above).
31. Report in *The Times*, March 1st 1984.
32. Neil Macfarlane, House of Commons, December 16th 1983.

GLOSSARY

Acromegaly Excessive secretion of growth hormone during adult-hood, the consequence of which is the growth of certain bones, especially those of the face.

Addison's disease A disorder characterised by adrenocortical insufficiency, i.e. the adrenal cortex fails to produce corticosteroids.

Adrenal glands Endocrine glands located above the kidneys. The middle part (medulla) secretes the hormones adrenalin and nor-adrenalin while the outer cortex produces corticosteroids.

Adrenalin (epinephrine) One of the hormones secreted by the adrenal glands at times of stress and fear.

Adrenocorticotrophic hormone (ACTH) A hormone produced by the pituitary gland in response to a releasing factor from the hypothalamus. ACTH stimulates the adrenal cortex to produce corticosteroids.

Amenorrhoea Cessation of menstrual periods which may be caused by a number of factors such as stress, regular excessive exercise, loss of body weight or old age.

Amphetamine A synthetic stimulant drug which elevates mood, increases arousal and curbs appetite. It acts by increasing the release of neurotransmitters, like dopamine and noradrenaline, in various brain regions.

Anabolic steroids Steroids which promote nitrogen retention and so aid the build-up of proteins. This may cause the development of bigger muscles.

Analgesics Drugs used to combat pain. They range from aspirin-like substances which prevent pain at source by reducing inflamma-

178

tion, to powerful opium–related drugs which act on the central nervous system to blur the perception of pain.

Androgens   The so-called male sex hormones. Testosterone is the principal mammalian androgen.

Androstenedione   An androgen secreted by the adrenal cortex of both males and females.

Anorectic drugs   Drugs used clinically to treat obesity by curbing appetite or enhancing satiety.

Beta-blockers   Drugs used clinically to treat cardiac disorders and high blood pressure. They are also used to reduce feelings of 'nerves' of 'stage fright' which occur as a result of activity in the sympathetic nervous system.

Blood-doping   The withdrawal and re-infusion of red blood cells in order to increase the oxygen-carrying capacity of the blood.

Central nervous system   The brain and spinal cord.

Cerebral cortex   The outer layer of the largest brain structure, the cerebrum.

Chromosomes   (see sex chromosomes)

Cocaine   A powerful stimulant and local anaesthetic drug found in Coca leaves.

Corticosteroids   Hormones released from the cortex of the adrenal glands during times of stress. The glucocorticoids (e.g. cortisol) increase glucose levels in the blood and have anti-inflammatory effects. The mineralocorticoids (e.g. aldosterone) increase the retention of salts.

Cushing's disease   Excessive secretion of steroids from the cortex of the adrenal gland.

Diuretics   Drugs which promote urine production.

Dopamine   A neurotransmitter in the brain; one of the catecholamines.

Doping   As defined by the IAAF: 'the use or distribution to an athlete of certain substances which could have the effect of improving artificially the athlete's physical and/or mental condition and so augment his athletic performance.'

Eleutherococcus   A plant, the extract of which has been used by some athletes as a stimulant.

Endocrine gland   A gland which secretes its hormones directly into the blood (the alternative type are exocrine which secrete their products elsewhere, e.g. the salivary glands).

Endorphins and enkephalins   The so-called endogenous opiates.

179

Substances produced in the central nervous system which have actions similar to those of morphine.

Ephedrine A stimulant drug originally extracted from species of the plant *Ephedra*.

Glucocorticoids (see Corticosteroids)

Gonadotrophins Complex chemicals released from the pituitary gland. They cause increased secretion of hormones from the gonads (ovaries and testes).

Growth hormone Also known as somatotrophin. Its principal action is on the long bones which elongate under its influence. Lack of it before puberty causes dwarfism in children, and excessive amounts results in gigantism.

Heroin An opiate otherwise known as diamorphine. It is an addictive analgesic with a potency 4 or 5 times that of morphine.

Hormones Substances produced in one part of the body then carried via the blood to affect one or more target organs in a different area.

Menstrual cycle The female reproductive cycle in primates (humans and apes) controlled by the secretion of gonadotrophins and ovarian hormones (oestrogens and progesterone).

Minerals Salts, e.g. sodium, potassium, calcium, iron, etc.

Mineralocorticoids (see Corticosteroids)

Narcotics In the USA this term refers to any addictive drug. Strictly speaking narcotics are central nervous system depressants that produce narcosis (from Greek, meaning stupor).

Nitrogen One of the components of amino acids, the building blocks that form proteins.

Noradrenalin One of the catecholamines; it is a hormone produced by the adrenal medulla and probably also acts as a neurotransmitter in the brain.

Oestrogen One of the ovarian hormones that control the female reproductive cycle. It is responsible for releasing eggs (ova) from the ovary.

Placebo A 'dummy' tablet or injection which often has powerful effects when the recipient believes he or she has been given a particular drug.

Progesterone An ovarian hormone which normally maintains the uterine lining, and also maintains the placenta (afterbirth) during pregnancy.

Prostaglandins Substances produced by the body at the site of injury; they cause inflammation and pain. Their synthesis is prevented by aspirin-like drugs.

Proteins Large, complex sequences of amino acids which have various functions throughout the body.

Puberty A time of dramatic hormonal fluctuations which mark the transition from childhood to adolescence.

Radioimmunoassay A technique for identifying certain biological chemicals.

Somatotrophin (see Growth hormone)

Stimulants General term for drugs which increase alertness and reduce fatigue.

Strychnine A stimulant extracted from the seeds of *Nux vomica*. It enhances spinal cord reflexes and in higher doses produces convulsions and death.

Sympathetic nervous system A branch of the involuntary or autonomic nervous system which is activated at times of fear, anger or stress.

Sympathomimetic amines Substances which produce effects similar to those seen after activation of the sympathetic nervous system. Many stimulants fall into this class of drugs.

Testosterone A gonadal hormone produced in large amounts by men and, to a lesser extent, by women. It has a powerful anabolic action but its primary role is to develop and maintain the male reproductive system.

Thyroid gland An endocrine gland in the neck which concentrates iodine and incorporates it into hormones such as thyroxine; these act as general metabolic stimulants.

Tranquillisers A diffuse class of drugs which have sedative properties. Certain of these are used in the treatment of schizophrenia and others in anxiety.

Vitamins A varied group of substances that organisms have to extract from their environment, usually through their diet. They are essential to life, hence their original name 'vital-amines'.

NAME INDEX

Abashdze, N.   15
Alen, M.   45, 131
Ali, M.   111
Altig, R.   7
Andersson, F.   133
Angus, R.   19, 20, 142
Anquetil, J.   7
Austin, T.   93

Balas, I.   75
Baldicheva, N.   11
Bannister, R.   43
Bautista, D.   115
Beckett, Prof.   27, 59, 62, 64, 114
Beecher, H.   23
Beeten, B.   139
Bello, B.   101
Bender, R.   86
Benning, C.   15, 50
Bertol, E.   115
Bertrand, M.   13
Birlenbach, H.   9
Blagoev, B.   167
Blair, S.   23
Blue, V.   169
Botham, I.   90
Bouton, J.   32
Bramble, L.   167
Brekhman, Prof.   108

Bresolles, P. (C).   76
Brooks, Prof.   12, 59, 61, 62
Browner, R.   31
Bruch, R.   53
Brundage, A.   6
Bull, M.   128

Cameron, M.   167
Capes, G.   45, 46, 62
Caula, L.   76
Chagnon, L.   16, 112
Chandler, J.   23
Charmis   2
Cioltan, V.   12
Ciorosion, D.   167
Clark, K.   87
Clarke, K.   96
Clarke, K., Dr.   139
Clarke, R.L.   135
Clausnitzer, C.   86
Coe, S.   1
Colorado, R.   99
Coleman, V.   93
Comaneci, N.   74
Connolly, H.   1, 12
Cook, T.   65
Cooper, N.   126, 138
Cowan, D.   65, 131

SUBJECT INDEX

187